# Inside Psychosis

This book offers an introductory overview of treatment of psychosis in inpatient acute ward settings, looking at both male and female wards.

Taking a broadly psychoanalytic perspective, the book explores the organisational dynamics on male and female acute wards, exploring both patient and staff dynamics. Containing detailed case studies from across male and female psychiatric wards in London, the author sets out how psychoanalytic concepts, such as transference, questions of trauma and issues of gender, can shape both the presentation of psychosis and our understanding and treatment of it. The book then explores the part played by religion in psychosis and equips readers with ideas for future practice and training on psychosis.

With clear guidance on how to understand and work with psychosis in an inpatient setting, and how many unconscious factors can affect patients and staff, this is key reading for psychiatrists, psychoanalysts and therapists, clinical psychologists and other mental health professionals working in inpatient acute care and community settings.

**Helen L. Holmes** is educated from Oxford University, UCL, Kings College London and Heythrop College, London. Helen is the Clinical Director of The Blues Clinic in London, working with children, adults, couples and families, from a diversity of backgrounds and cultures. She practices as a psychoanalyst, forensic psychodynamic psychotherapist, family and couples practitioner, accredited Autism and ADHD assessor, accredited mediator and clinical supervisor. Helen has written and taught psychology-related courses at LSE and Birkbeck College and innovated a popular clinical project about adolescent self-harm cessation at IOPPN, King's College London.

'*Inside Psychosis* is based on Helen L. Holmes' work over a period of 15 years with deeply disturbed patients. She recognises the profound need of these individuals to be listened to in a safe relationship of genuine professional trust and care. Though her primary lens is psychoanalytic she does not hesitate to use a variety of therapeutic perspectives such as cognitive behavior therapy or the person-centered approach. Given the importance of religion and spirituality for many patients, the author advocates a bio psychosocial model of schizophrenia, that should encompass the spiritual needs of patients. Holmes succeeds wonderfully to demystify schizophrenia and psychosis and thus lessen fear and myths about these terrifying conditions. This book will be of great assistance to both, health professionals dealing with people suffering of schizophrenia and the patients so diagnosed, their families and friends. Highly recommended.'

**Thomas R. Verny MD**, *DHL (Hon), DPsych, FRCPC, FAPA, Founding President APPPAH, Author of* The Secret Life of the Unborn Child *with John Kelly,* Pre-Parenting *with Pamela Weintraub, and* The Embodied Mind.

'Helen L. Holmes' *Inside Psychosis* is a brave and engagingly written mosaic of many of the extraordinary complexities that arise within the interrelations between serious talking and profound listening both in the therapeutic situation and in supervision. Holmes' lengthy and wide-ranging experience in a variety of clinical settings, and with diverse treatment modalities, make this book an important read for anyone wishing to learn about the intimate detail of the internal worlds of psychotic patients, and the psychotic elements in us all. Despite the horrors it details, it is a strangely uplifting book. At the end of the day, as Holmes' work illustrates, the talking/listening 'cures' are treatments of love.'

**Richard Ekins,** *retired member of the British Psychoanalytical Society and Emeritus Professor of Sociology and Cultural Studies, Ulster University, UK*

'One of the delights of having been involved in Higher Education is seeing former students make their mark in their chosen areas, developing expertise and scholarship that go far beyond anything one might have been able to teach them. That is certainly my response, as a retired teacher of psychology of religion in the University of London, to reading Helen L. Holmes' new book, *Inside Psychosis*.

In the course of many years of mainly one-to-one work with a great variety of people living with and dealing with the experience of psychosis, Helen has come to a near-unique understanding of the different factors involved, and of the range of explanatory models that have been formulated in the attempt to comprehend, and to work with and for, such individuals.

*Inside Psychosis* takes the reader into this complex world, managing to convey something of the experience of individuals experiencing schizophrenia and psychosis, as well as surveying the theoretical and professional discussions that are slowly shedding light on what has all too easily been seen as requiring treatment only with medication. Religious and spiritual elements are frequently present in psychotic and other schizophrenic experiences, and *Inside Psychosis* explores the multiple differences involved. These include how some cultures regard as "normal" and indeed significant what others regard as pathological, and how western medicine has found it almost impossible to include religion and spirituality in any attempted whole-person approaches to patient care.

Helen L. Holmes' book, in its combination of theoretical discussion and case studies, brings together lived experience and disciplined reflection: it is educative not just of the understanding, but of the heart.'

**Revd Brendan Callaghan SJ, MA, MPhil, MTh, Hon FCP,** *Formerly University of London, Senior Lecturer in the Psychology of Religion, Principal of Heythrop College, University of Oxford: Master of Campion Hall, Institute of Medical Ethics: General Secretary*

# Inside Psychosis

A clinical and therapeutic exploration of working on male and female acute psychiatric wards

**Helen L. Holmes**

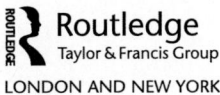
Routledge
Taylor & Francis Group

LONDON AND NEW YORK

Designed cover image: Abstract Aerial Art © Getty

First published 2025
by Routledge
4 Park Square, Milton Park, Abingdon, Oxon OX14 4RN

and by Routledge
605 Third Avenue, New York, NY 10158

*Routledge is an imprint of the Taylor & Francis Group, an informa business*

*British Library Cataloguing-in-Publication Data*
A catalogue record for this book is available from the British Library

ISBN: 978-1-032-83376-7 (hbk)
ISBN: 978-1-032-83228-9 (pbk)
ISBN: 978-1-003-50905-9 (ebk)

DOI: 10.4324/9781003509059

Typeset in Optima
by Apex CoVantage, LLC

To my dearest mother, father and two brothers, with much love and thanks.

# Contents

*'Though this be madness, yet there is method in't'.*
**Hamlet, Act II, Scene II – William Shakespeare**

# Foreword

This book takes a position on the unresolved question of how far distant psychosis is from ordinary experiences we have of the world and of our own selves. Down through history, it has mostly been taken that the distance is unbridgeable. However, some, including psychodynamic therapists, have introduced us to the possibility that we are nearer than we think. Helen L. Holmes' book is written with an impassioned enthusiasm that attempts a much closer, almost 'inside', experience of a 'psychotic' state of mind.

This describes the personal voyages of a number of people Holmes has offered treatment to. The close descriptions of the many topics give a wide panorama of the field, from the very general features of what is called psychosis to the small details of the personal experiences of each case. Everything is refocused in ordinary language. So we have the privilege of entering the author's wide and devoted experience of a whole zone of our human world most of us have tended to avoid since history began.

And it also gives us the privilege looking at, and sympathising with, the sufferers' experiences of themselves. It is an act of devotion to attend and re-attend to the horrors that engage them, a devotion not only of the author but also of the reader who will enter these disabling experiences of our fellow persons. This is an opportunity to survey this map of troubled experiences without having to travel too deeply into the territory ourselves. It goes a long way to de-mythologise the thinking and experiencing of psychotic states of mind.

We are, most of us, willing to explore different states of mind. There are so many of us who automatically assume we know the experiences of other species of animals, such as cats, dogs and horses, but we run from an acquaintance with what life is like for these fellow human beings we label 'psychotic'. In many circumstances, we like to alter our mental state with an occasional gin and tonic or a pint of export. Indeed, even watching a thriller on television or a romantic opera or a bit of pornography are ways of coaxing ourselves into different forms of understanding and familiarity with various states of our conscious awareness. These unreal journeys of our minds are not so different from where these people go in their psychotic states. Of course, our willing exploration is likely to be less far-reaching than those unreal journeys that people take when they enter a psychotic period. We can bring ourselves back after we switch off the television or leave the theatre or concert hall. And indeed, some of our mental health professionals today are not so happy with the distancing approach based solely on medication.

So should we really open the dustbin and dump out of our minds the madness that can exist there? Is it really so dangerous? Of course, human empathy has its limits, like everything else. But can we stop rejecting an awareness of their world and then carefully join with these unfortunate others, or could we only listen to King Lear's desperation soliloquies in staged performances? This book offers us an opportunity to come close to psychotic states without a concern we might step beyond the limits that we normally patrol. What can be gained is that we see even the worst of experiences may not be so threatening as the sufferers imply and as we so easily believe. Once communicated and listened to, we can recognise they are probably ordinary human experiences which, though terrifying some of us, are not so different from the anxieties, grief, guilt and conflict most of us have faced.

It is impressive that the willingness to consider the actual experiences of people in psychotic states will lead to their actually telling their experiences to us. Despite the frequent reference to the 'talking cure', it must, as we all know, be a *listening* cure.

The author is very clear that there is another half to the process of listening: to listen to oneself at the same time, listening to one's own reactions at every point during the connection. One can only make contact with people in psychotic states by making human contact with one's own personal experience as a human person. It is as if the humanity concealed behind a psychotic state can detect when you are there with yourself and with them. And moreover, it becomes a prologue to the patient being able to listen to *them*selves.

The psychodynamic approach to schizophrenia appears to be unusually difficult because the understanding of the unconscious processes does not lead directly to a mode of intervention. Perhaps this is because, usually in a psychodynamic therapy, an understanding unconscious processes leads directly to bringing that understanding to consciousness. With psychotic processes, the problem is different. It is not that the unconscious is concealed and a therapist must engage in a struggle to bring the concealed into the open. Instead, there is little of the unconscious concealed; rather, it is the reality out there that is concealed. Instead of opening the person to what they are concealing from themselves, the psychotic needs the real world to exist for them, in all its painful aspects. As a result, there should be a need to focus on the real world first before diving into a deep unconscious. Helen L. Holmes has presented a therapeutic approach which starts just there; the therapist will conduct a patient-centred approach, which engages with the *patient's* perception of reality. It is a confirmation that, in reality, the therapist has heard exactly what the patient says. A repetition of their own words could almost be a reassurance. And *it is*, in a sense, a reassurance; reality is not an engagement with a separate other. Rather, the therapist is a reality that models their self as it connects with the other who *expresses* their self for them.

Particularly with her last case, Melanie, Helen L. Holmes then describes how it can be possible to move on from this first step. The second step is an approach to a more conventional psychodynamic separateness in which the therapist becomes a perceiving other, struggling with a curiosity about something unknown. The contrast is towards a discovery rather than reassurance of what is already believed.

*Inside Psychosis* is an invaluable account if we wish to come closer to these persons extruded from ordinary life. It has been heartening to read of the adventure of someone willing to journey amongst the experience most of us shy away from. Anyone who has a relative or friend who is cursed with such a medical diagnosis will be helpfully informed. It should reassure professionals with a career that has avoided close encounters by using medical drugs to simulate a caring practice. This book presents therapists, mental health professionals and the troubled public with an insight into facing the challenge of these most difficult problems.

Bob Hinshelwood
August 2024

# Acknowledgements

There is one author of this book but so many other authors who need to be acknowledged. Initially, enormous gratitude is due to my parents who have supported and encouraged me consistently and generously in my life and through my education and trainings, with good humour. My mother is just as avid a learner as me and offered me the invaluable insight early on in my life to get to know myself by getting to know others who are different from me. I took this to heart and explored many other cultures by travelling, reading and setting up different inter-cultural groups. My mother's sense of humour and consistent encouragement of me has been invaluable, inspiring me to explore the world and learn from many different cultures and religions, facilitating my growth and development immensely. As with my mother, my father's highly astute thinking and empowering approach towards me has helped me navigate life; thank you does not adequately convey my gratitude for all that they have given me. Heartfelt thanks are additionally due to my dearest brothers – one elder, one younger – both of whom continue to greatly inspire and encourage me in my life with their ingenuity, experiences, insights, love, humour and creativity. I am very grateful and lucky to have had the good fortune of such brothers in my life. My maternal grandmother, Jenny, was a great source of strength for me, encouraging me to keep on writing. My mother's sister Jean and my uncle Gerry Wheale have always been supportive of me, for which I have been greatly heartened and grateful from early childhood. My father's brother William Holmes, an Oxford English scholar and Shakespearean actor, is sorely missed for his sharp wit, people observations and life tips, with whom our family were close. Thank you to uncle Keith Scott, who studied Asian Studies at Oxford University and whose brilliant mind and teaching of Chinese continues to inspire me, alongside his quiet yet shrewd manner and kindness. Uncle Malcolm Scott has shared much with our family in heartfelt and humorous ways, and I want to show my appreciation of him here.

Heartfelt thanks are certainly due to Heythrop College, University of London, for a mind-opening and invaluable education base in philosophy, theology, psychology of religion, interreligious dialogue and so much more.

I could not have wanted for a better education than this, by developing and deepening my thinking, my eyes and mind were opened. I am fortunate to have been encouraged by my prior tutor Reverend Brendan Callaghan to explore the psychology of religion, taking me around the world researching religious communities, presenting and publishing my findings and reflections. Reverend Michael Barnes helped me to understand better street level diversity in Southall and beyond, which remains invaluable and for which I am deeply grateful. Reverend Nick King has offered me opportunity, hope and deep understanding, which I can't thank him enough for, this has been life-giving. For these opportunities and the understanding shown, I am eternally and sincerely grateful. Thanks also are due to University College London and Oxford University, where I completed important clinical trainings, which I have managed to use to help people in need.

Importantly, many thanks to the Routledge commissioning editors who supported this project and to whom I owe my gratitude. Furthermore, of enormous importance are the multitude of patients on acute wards and in the community, with whom I am utterly privileged to have shared in their lives and to listen to their experiences for over 17 years. I recall late evenings when the nurses instructed me off the ward and I tore myself away from this remarkable and unique learning experience for in-depth understanding of the inner workings of the psyche to catch the last bus home across London. Ward life was of such rich interest to me, in relation to observing the manifestations of the adult mind in crisis, offering me glimpses of inner psychic life. It remains such an invaluable experience to have closely listened to and shared in the lives of these remarkable and extremely vulnerable men and women and, at times, their families. I want to heartily and warmly thank each and every individual for sharing their experiences with me, often very tragic and painful, but nonetheless we sat, talked, cried, ate, created and laughed together, seeking threads of hope through very dark times. Working on wards is a profound and privileged experience.

Being permitted access to the wards at each hospital, in both paid and unpaid capacities, would not have been possible without the support of the hospital and ward staff, who recognised my burgeoning desire to better understand the mind in crisis and then try to work out what would help these individuals who are so profoundly marginalised, pushed to the peripheries of society and living with more than horrible day-to-day internal experiences, little understood by the majority, including the individuals. We need to try to understand better and reduce this persistent suffering, facilitating expression of their otherwise isolated worlds. Thankfully, over the years, I have gathered insights and practical points that may help. On various wards, I sometimes sat on seven-hour long, weekly ward rounds, alongside supporting the individuals living as inpatients there, with chronic conditions within the psychoses and schizophrenias. I hope that I was careful enough to tread lightly and sensitively into their fragile, temporary ward living space; thank you to all the patients and staff, your lives and work are heart-rendering.

I would like to thank Dr. John Steiner, an eminent psychiatrist and psychoanalyst. Dr. John Steiner showed me how he is on the side of the patient, aligning with my perspective. Furthermore, he further showed me great sensitivity, understanding and kindness, which I will never forget. I was surprised and delighted to be invited to take over the therapy group on one of the female wards by a consultant psychiatrist and psychoanalyst, which he had been running for some years and which I then happily facilitated for many years following, offering women and then men a safe space to share about their lives whilst engaging in creative activities and themed discussions, all chosen by the group members. Nonetheless, I needed to stay alert to change moods and manage sometimes rapidly shifting perceptions, including potential and actual coercion, aggression, violence and manipulation.

I can't thank the ward manager enough for his insights, consistent support and kindness, whose ward I volunteered on for nearly six years and who I saw as consistently compassionate and humane towards the women on the ward. He showed time and again that calmly being alongside patients and speaking quietly, clearly and respectfully works well. Many thanks to the ward staff for understanding and responding to my enthusiasm for learning about psychosis. Sincere and heartfelt thanks go to all the ward managers and nurses with whom I enjoyed working closely throughout the years and for the wealth of opportunity to gain understanding and learn about what helps individuals in the process of psychosis. I have been enabled to take what I have learned on acute wards into my current private practice and clinic, where I am proudly well-equipped to help the most vulnerable in our communities towards a better quality of life, who are sadly often turned away by most other clinicians. I offer a welcome, safe and confidential space, where individuals, couples and families can think with me about what is troubling them. I am equipped, at this point in my life, to work with both more common and severe mental health difficulties, and I am thankful for my multi-disciplinary team's support.

A huge thank you is necessary to Professor Robert Hinshelwood, who initiated, encouraged and supervised my clinical work with adults on acute wards for 17 years (2007–2024). He helped me to think about the organisational dynamics on wards and the psychoanalytic processes of those presenting with the psychoses and schizophrenias, with whom I worked therapeutically. Professor Hinshelwood has greatly enhanced my understanding and therapeutic treatment of those experiencing psychosis, helping me to help numerous individuals to better understand themselves and towards a significantly improved quality of life for themselves. My work with Professor Hinshelwood continues now beyond his supervision, as I hope to have taken in and reflected on his speculations, and it continues to be a marvel how he has such in-depth insight into the workings of individuals, in these acute states of mind.

Thanks are definitely due to Dr. Duncan McLean, who supervised my work for five years, with families and individuals with a range of difficulties alongside psychosis, non-epileptic seizures, schizophrenia and personality difficulties, helping me to develop understanding alongside a plethora of new therapeutic skills to assist forward those living with inordinate amounts of distress and pain. I learned a great deal, for which I am very grateful.

Additionally, many thanks to Dr. Nancy Burke, a psychoanalyst in the USA, who also supervises my clinical work with individuals experiencing psychosis, offering me such valuable psychodynamic insights which helped patients' lives progress well; I really cannot thank her enough. I would further like to warmly thank Dr. Constanza Aranguren, who is another talented psychoanalyst and supervisor, a compassionate human being and who has supported my work with patients with insightful and kind clinical supervision. Dr. Anthony Roberts (now sadly deceased) introduced me to DSM-IV in 2007 and was a consistently enormous source of inspiration with my clinical work with children, adolescents and their families, for which I cannot possibly find adequate words to thank him enough. There are many other stars with whom I have worked closely, who have offered me encouragement and support in my endeavours for justice and fairness – namely, Jeremy Oliver, whose astuteness, professionalism, capacity for concern and adherence to social justice led to good overcoming evil. I can't thank him enough, lifelong. I inherited from my parents and grandparents a strong commitment to helping the most marginalised, the most vulnerable, towards having a more equal opportunity to rise and a better quality of life. I sincerely apologise if I have overlooked anyone here. I offer my deep gratitude to all the gems with whom I have worked with and learned so much from.

# Preface

My interest in people was a fascination for me from an early age, as I wondered about myself in relation to family members and was encouraged to read widely by my parents. Having studied a range of six humanities subjects at A level, including Philosophy and Psychology, I then studied Law Politics and English, then Philosophy and Theology. Philosophy and psychology are closely interrelated in many of the philosophical areas of interest in life, and having completed my studies, I helped set up the *Big Issue* in London, where I encountered psychosis in especially young street homeless people for the first time, who were living in cardboard boxes whilst taking a range of prescribed and unprescribed uppers and downers to cope with their exposure to the elements. These individuals were part of a street community, and they shared about the varied reasons leading to living on the streets. Working with addiction and insecurity, sex work and the difficulties of being housed within four walls – along with the loneliness and isolation this brought in contrast to living amongst a street fraternity offering belonging – was illuminating. I studied Psychology of religion at Heythrop College London, and my dissertation about pre- and perinatal religious development took off at a great surprise to me in the USA and UK, published later as a book in 2020: *Seeing God in our birth experiences: A psychoanalytic inquiry into pre and perinatal religious development* (Routledge Studies in Religion). I was fortunate to have further benefited enormously from Reverend Michael Barnes' teaching on interfaith; then setting up and facilitating a Muslim and non-Muslim women's dialogue group for many years.

I had travelled the world single-handedly researching religious communities, taking me out of my comfort zone, as I braved the Rockies for personal development, following in the steps of Simone de Beauvoir. Like Freud, I have a lifelong interest in religion and in understanding why religion, in all its ramifications. These are deeply personal matters. A deep understanding of myself in relation to others has been one of the most empowering life processes for me, leading to independence in relation to others. I have continued studying to better inform myself and to improve as a person and professional and have no regrets about spending the majority of my life on acute psychiatric wards with children, adolescents and adults, listening also to parents and families. There is much pain in the world, and with insight, the suffering advances the person as a human being, in my opinion. Without insight and a want to understand further, harm can often be caused. Another major learning experience was when I underwent a two-year infant observation which was central to developing my analytic stance. Working with individuals with severe mental health difficulties has become my lifelong commitment, creating equal opportunities to rise and bringing about justice. I will continue learning and putting my learning into practice to help those in most need. It is extremely important to me that the marginalised are understood and brought to safety through consistent safe and reliable relationships. There is much work to be done, and the more people involved, the more lives can start to be transformed. Everyone deserves, at least, a sense of belonging. We *all* have so much that is constructive to contribute to life, in myriad ways.

This book breaks new ground in relation to narrating therapeutic work with individuals with psychosis, mainly from the psychoanalytic perspective, the thinkers of which tradition remain remarkably thoughtful and insightful. For example, Professor Robert Hinshelwood, Herbert Rosenfeld, Henri Rey, John Steiner and Isobel Menzies-Lyth (regarding organisational dynamics). However, different modalities are also included, namely, the systemic approaches, alongside that of cognitive-behavioural therapy and the humanistic person-centred school when offering therapy in secure mental health institutions. I want to demonstrate that whichever training one has undergone, skills can be used to help those suffering abominable states of mind to feel less distressed, unwanted and isolated. I think clinicians need confidence to work with individuals with psychosis and schizophrenia. It starts with being able to be in the same room as an individual suffering so deeply, to be able to overcome all manner of feeling and prejudices and to reach out as one human to another as safe, consistent and reliable practitioners.

This account attempts to describe and offer my thinking about experiences observed over a period of 17 years, whilst working on acute, inpatient psychiatric wards in London. The essential importance of listening to one another is perhaps very much lost in contemporary culture, perhaps as a result of such competitive individualism, social media and quick-fix cures, which bypass a proper concern for each other. We all need to be heard whilst growing up through childhood and adolescence, but I question to what extent people actually feel listened to and whether what is said is considered of value. If we lack being heard in everyday life, then imagine what it is like for those suffering with the psychoses. These individuals are often lucky if someone says hello to them, creating such a hunger to be seen and heard with respect and value, rather than being left with the repeated experience of abandonment, suspicion, fear and hatred. I recognise the basic and profound need of these individuals to be listened to in safe relationships of genuine professional trust and care.

A further main aim is a movement from learning from experience to try to demystify the psychoses in order to lessen fear and myths about these terrifying states of mind through writing about my understanding of real-life encounters with men and women on acute psychiatric wards. In my presentations of all the people I have gratefully met and worked with in therapy, account has been made of my own social constructions affecting my perceptions, alongside self-reflection on the processes involved in my choice of words as possible countertransference, for which I take full responsibility for. Countertransference, describes the often unconscious communications from the patient to the clinician, which, when recognised and reflected upon, can inform what is going on at the core of the patient – what needs to be confronted and perhaps can't be spoken about by the patient, of which they are unaware. Transference refers to the patient's unresolved thoughts, feelings, desires and memories from past experiences and relationships, becoming projected in and onto the therapist in the present. Recognising transference and countertransference mechanisms at play offers the unique opportunity to work through the patient's experiences safely with the therapist to a more resolved state of mind and being.

It has been a great privilege to have been able to share in so many individuals' lives on these inpatient wards, and to genuinely engage their trust has been one of the most fulfilling experiences of my life. As stated previously, I valued my ward visits so much that I had to tear myself away, sometimes after 12 hours of deliberate weekend volunteering, when most inpatients were more isolated due to the lack of ward activities and/or visits from friends, family or professionals. It has been a mix of truly fascinating, moving and distressing experiences to witness such a range of presentations on the wards, mostly involving individuals in significant crisis in their lives – matters of life and death. I am thankful to have felt and feel very well supported in myself, having undergone a full analysis. Additionally, I have diligently and consistently undergone ongoing continuing personal and professional development as a learner, including numerous trainings, seminars, reading and reflection, and I am considered to have done more than most, to better equip myself to help the most vulnerable in our communities. I feel fortunate in the way that I have received solid support from ward staff but also in clinical supervision and my personal life. My motivation for working in both paid and voluntary capacities for many years has been fueled with a curiosity to better understand the experiences of those who have been diagnosed with severe mental health conditions, such as the schizophrenias and psychoses, and others, such as eating disorders and addictions. It seems that trauma pervades all conditions and I work with carefully.

One of the main aims of this book is to show that significant therapeutic work can be progressed with individuals, diagnosed or not, with identified schizophrenia and psychosis. Although my therapeutic and analytic base modality as a psychotherapist is psychoanalytic, I have ventured to learn different therapeutic perspectives and drawn upon these in relation to assisting individuals with psychosis to demonstrate that at least the psychoanalytic (already well established as an appropriate approach to understanding psychosis, which may need to be modified due to the possible fragility of the patient), systemic and family approaches, cognitive-behavioural therapy (such as for cognitive input regarding the detrimental effects on cognition via medication), mentalisation-based therapy for encouraging awareness of other minds and empathy and the person-centred approach when working on wards. Many individuals with the psychoses need therapists who are equipped to work with them to improve their condition and lives. I feel at a great disadvantage since I don't have any personal experience of the symptoms of psychosis or schizophrenia, and I still venture to understand two of the main aspects of schizophrenia: 1) paranoia and 2) memory, which have been highlighted as the key areas needing much more understanding from a patient perspective. Paranoid experiences, unfortunately, by their very nature, seem to obstruct sharing about them, almost like the individual becomes trapped in a paranoid construction and is silenced. I need to think more about how paranoia leads to delusions and the interpretations these interpretations can foster into terrifying states of mind. I regret, in a way, not having personal experience to enable me to gain insight into psychosis and schizophrenia to help these individuals more. I consider that clinicians need webinars on lived experience to better understand the experience they have not encountered themselves, apart from through observation and books.

The array of medications that many individuals take daily, often leaves them in a comatose state, whilst drug companies earn billions. How can this be an ethical situation, and why has medical know-how not produced safer medications that enable life rather than limit it? Perhaps we all need to share in not knowing enough about the brain to be able to understand the psychoses well enough. Perhaps the new drug for schizophrenia from the USA, KarXT, would help. It is designed to reduce positive and negative symptoms of schizophrenia, with fewer side effects than other anti-psychotic medications create, such as weight gain and diabetes (Barnes, 2024). Let's see what patients say about it.

It is of paramount importance to iterate that all individuals have given written informed consent for their material to be included in this book which they read first and were asked for any changes, following a thorough assessment regarding their capacity to give such consent. All identifying features have been anonymised in respect of protecting their privacy and confidentiality. All individuals have generously encouraged material about them to be published in the hope that learning about psychosis and schizophrenia is inspired.

All correspondence with the author, please send to helenholmes009@ gmail.com, with thanks. Let's start a conversation.

# Introduction

From observation and learning from experience, it seems that an unsettling and curious situation presents itself when raising the subject of schizophrenia and psychosis, such that these words, almost onomatopoeically, appear to create conflicted responses within us, preventing us from seeing the person. There is something perhaps presumptive in using such terms to define another, creating a potentially highly unbalanced power dynamic of the psychiatrist/ team, evoking further fear in already paranoid and vulnerable individuals from diverse backgrounds, cultures, displaced and traumatic situations. For example, there are far too many clinicians in ward rounds. My main observation is that the power dynamics in psychiatric hospitals needs to be redressed to achieve a more humane balance. Patients know more about their experiences than most psychiatrists, who have mainly gained their knowledge from books. It seems that there is almost a taboo around discussing schizophrenia and psychosis, possibly born from a fear of recognising the symptoms in oneself, without being easily able to grasp a clear understanding of what schizophrenia and psychosis looks or feels like. The possible difficulty in being able to grasp what schizophrenia and psychosis are like, apart from for those who have family members with such diagnoses and/or professional experience, seems to be that the collection of symptoms named schizophrenia is not perhaps as certain or clearly defined as we may wish or expect from DSM-IV/V (American Psychiatric Association, 1994, 2013) and beyond. Working with individuals and families, where a diagnosis of psychosis or schizophrenia has been given, it seems that in private practice, I have been more able to work supportively with a gentle counselling approach and become increasingly psychodynamic or psychoanalytic as the individual's ego is strengthened. However, in mental health institutions, I have tended to adopt a more person-centred approach, in relation to the perceived fragility of the individuals in crisis, often having recently survived a reported paranoid massive attack on their own minds and bodies.

The terms schizophrenia and psychosis seem to erect a screen beyond which most don't manage to explore and, therefore, understand or challenge their meaning. From my substantial experience of working closely with individuals with these diagnoses, I think that most, if not all, would likely not be in the situation they are in if they had gained safe, consistent and reliable

DOI: 10.4324/9781003509059-1

attention to their needs in all senses as they were raised. It seems they are struggling with an unstable and dysregulated sense of self. The medication seems to replace what parents, often at no fault of theirs, couldn't offer but can be sorely needed. A main problem appears to be inconsistent and unreliable caregiving. A trauma-informed approach, which seeks to acknowledge, without judgement, the transgenerational transmission of trauma in relation to the psychoses and schizophrenias, would likely help. Blame is not intended to be apportioned to parents who have an impossible task and have their own parenting to contend with, but as parents, we need to be *much* more aware of what we are transmitting to our offspring, who look to us as models and are dependent on our care. Perhaps a main difficulty is whether the situation can be thought about, often far too painful for this, or perceived as far too painful with inadequate support or unconscious or conscious forbiddance. Currently, many individuals are being re-diagnosed with PTSD or complex trauma to replace schizophrenia, as is known. One can wonder about the function of psychosis in families, perhaps keeping the family together, or as a way for parents not to take responsibility for their own hurts communicated via their parenting, such as when sexual abuse has occurred.

We are aware that it takes a lot of psychic work to come to realise that there is so much about the human brain and mind that we don't currently understand and perhaps may never understand. Just as GPs may not really know what the cause of the seemingly physical symptoms are apart from a likely virus, perhaps our need for someone medically trained to 'know' definitively stems from the understandable human difficulty in tolerating uncertainty and the unpleasant accompanying feelings of untethered anxiety. We possibly refer to a higher source of authority and 'knowledge' to help us cope with not knowing ourselves how to understand family and friends, who start behaving in ways that are unusual and perhaps frightening and dangerous to themselves and others. Importantly, in psychoanalytic parlance, our countertransference in relation to working one to one with individuals and their families gives us a direct felt sense of what is being communicated non-verbally, crucial for understanding of the core issues that the person needs to confront and the meaning of the resonance between the countertransference and, for example, family practices.

I notice that I work with the person-centred approach with individuals with psychosis in institutions and the psychoanalytic/psychodynamic approach in private practice. Mental health institutions hold great distress and fragility, and the psychoanalytic approach may arouse too much in an already very unsettled individual. However, the psychoanalytic stance offers much for inpatient therapy work, as observational and holding attitudes foster a space to think. This approach, alongside paying attention to our countertransference and focusing on moment-to-moment occurrences, reveals much about the patient without words. Once individuals reach the consulting room of a private clinic, they are usually functioning at a very different level than when they are in the hospital at the acute end of a crisis, where hospital staff and medication can bind the person together when they may be falling apart.

# 1 Clinical approach to therapy on acute psychiatric wards

'He had none: His flight was madness: when our actions do not, Our fears do make us traitors'.

*Macbeth*, Act IV, Scene II, Line 3 – William Shakespeare

When first working on psychiatric wards in London, I was struck by how individuals with psychosis, at times, communicated in ways that were difficult to decipher, such as hiding in cupboards, holding unusual bodily postures for long periods of time, thinking that they are Jesus or, most frequently, related to the Royal Family, screaming at others, talking loudly to themselves in full lively dialogue, fearing stabbing themselves in the stomach and various other dangerous and unusual acts that would understandably bring them to hospital. However, if I asked these individuals a normal question, such as 'What is your name?' 'How old are you?' 'Would you like to talk with me?' more often than not, such straightforward communications seemed to connect with a normal aspect of themselves, which started the relationship from seeming disordered thinking to a grounded conversation. This indicates to me a show of a kind of habit-forming madness which can be let to run on by the patient, staff, family and friends, unless we realise that there is a more normal aspect of the person which can be frequently easily accessed. For example, I observed a young man of around 26 years old making highly expressive, lively physical movements. I knew that he was interested in sports and asked, 'Would you like to have a conversation about sports?' He immediately switched out of the, one could describe perhaps as bizarre presentation, and responded yes. He and I went and talked together for over half an hour in a logical back-and-forth conversation. This example indicates that, perhaps, the logical self is hidden beneath a more bizarre presentation, which, if accepted, could fool us that logic nowhere exists in the person, when on exploration it does. Numerous times, I have found this to be the case with different individuals displaying what appears to be unusual behaviours. Perhaps the outward expression performs a function, enabling the individual to separate from others in the hospital, to keep their pain and distress at a distance alongside others, or to gain the help needed, alongside a plethora of other possible reasons.

DOI: 10.4324/9781003509059-2

Numerous times, when people on wards were speaking at 100mph, perhaps in a manic state and/or having taken some recreational drug, such as cocaine or amphetamine, it took me to persistently, assertively and kindly speak to the rational aspect of the individual and maintain my line of rational conversation to almost persuade them to safely come down, then start to engage in a much more back-and-forth ordinary conversation. It's like kindly and firmly bringing the person down from a lonely, overwhelmed emotional high to a more real and grounded place, where the person is helped to tolerate the disappointment of facing themselves and their environment – finding it tolerable, though relatively boring, but safe. It's like taking command of the situation and chipping away as a stone mason would but more gently, using logic to bring the person onto the same wavelength as me, and then talking about food, water, exercise and sleep. I have engaged with individuals with psychosis in therapy who are offered the boundaries they seem to need in order to contain the psychosis but who reject this since they prefer the interest and drama of the psychosis, being more freed up. Paying attention to and reading non-verbal communication is, therefore, very important. By taking control of the situation and offering a sense of safety to often frightened individuals who appear grandiose, one can help bring them into contact with reality in the relationship. However, the therapist needs to have worked through their own fears and anxieties to be able to be solid, relaxed and present for individuals experiencing psychosis.

Numerous times, I have sat next to a person clearly in great distress in one form or another, and the act of not appearing to be afraid by sitting next to them, not only conveyed that they are not alone but also that I can manage this and I won't be intimidated by this currently dominating aspect of their personality, appearing to move the person way out of control. Self-protection is necessary, but I have only been involved in one incident on a ward/community in over 32 years, where an individual threw a cup of urine over me before even speaking a first word to each other – some hello! Nurses huddled in the nursing station, peered out through the windows and then came and hugged and congratulated me for managing to bring another patient down to earth, perhaps as one of the medications would but in human form. I have also witnessed numerous times nurses and medical staff ignoring patients' knocks on the nursing station door, then inevitably seeing individuals kick off dangerously. We need to think what is being played out by the staff in such instances. Isabel Menzies-Lyth put forward her conjectures in relation to social structures as means of coping or mechanisms of defense; in effect, these are ways that staff working on wards avoid experiencing emotions, for example, anxiety, guilt and doubt. Menzies-Lyth offers invaluable insights as a Kleinian and Bionian psychoanalyst, and her writings span over 30 years of research, but this doesn't mean that further insight can't be gained. In one of her significant papers, Menzies-Lyth considered that the organisation of the nursing profession inadequately contains the extreme levels of anxiety and stress that nurses are exposed to and experience on long shifts on a daily basis (Menzies-Lyth, 1988).

I recall being asked to supervise a patient who was covered in faeces and very aggressive (frightened). Yet my intuition communicated that she was terrified beneath the frightening façade. By speaking with her frightened part, as one would gently and in a reassuring tone, she allowed me to run a bath for her and supervise her while she lay in an ever-increasing brown bath. She was literally bathing in her own shit, and I accepted her non-verbal demonstration of this. I suggested that we change the water so that she could become physically clean but quickly backed down when she insisted not. I stayed with her and made no further comment but ensured that she remained safe. This woman tried to bully me out of the bathroom, but I had been asked to supervise her and quietly but firmly stood my ground; she quietened and started sharing her thoughts with me. I was touched. She then wanted five more baths and eventually became clean. After which, she thanked me for helping her bathe, there being much reduced aggression in her voice then, as she had been allowed to take control of the situation, within a safe framework. The nurses had told me to tell her what to do and, if she didn't do it, tell her she can't have a bath. However, I allowed her to have numerous baths, and she calmed, perhaps by having some monitored power offered to her. I was observant in following the processes moment by moment, remaining open to what might work. It is always consistent kindness that touches these frequently frightened and confused souls. However, psychosis also needs a firm approach.

For example, on another psychosis ward, a young male patient remained in his room, lying on the floor day after day. It was discussed in the ward round that there needed to be a plan to help him out of his bedroom to engage more with others, apart from just eating. The plan was discussed with the man, and all appeared to be agreed, but when the hour came for him to leave his bedroom on the ward, which would then be locked for three to four hours, he appeared to be either asleep and unable to be woken, absent from his room, or in the shower at that particular time. This led to further interventions needed by the staff: to wake him, wait for him to finish his shower and for him to dress, or on some occasions to be located on the ward. At times, bank staff would let him onto the grounds, unaware of his plan. The staff needed to be very firm with this man, who wanted to ultimately remain in his room, maintaining the 'status quo'. But once he was locked out of his bedroom, he found plenty to do – a changed person, one could say, or a different version of himself than the one seen up to that point. If left, this man would never be discharged; he had, in effect, taken up residence in the unit.

One may assume that individuals on wards would want to leave, but we all get comfortable and can dislike change. Another patient reported acting on the voices of three ministers in his mind, each arguing with the others, each claiming to be right. This man was fairly elderly and single. I wondered if the three voices offered some companionship for him and that it would be quite unethical to take the voices away from him. What would he have then? After a year on the ward, it was posed to him that he would be discharged, which met with an understandably pronounced fearful response from him. This took a lot of careful work to increase his independence in preparation for moving to secure, sheltered accommodation. I learned a great deal from this process about dependency needs.

On a psychiatric ward, having engaged with an individual and established and started to gently but progressively build trust, through being consistent in every way possible, then individuals in crisis and with psychosis in this context, start to feel safer, and is a real achievement to see clients relaxing and becoming more trustful – a step towards humanity. Due to their understandably desperate need for someone to help them, this genuine trustworthiness is a lifeline to them. This is perhaps due to all the sensitivities of dependency needs and attachment, where the main priority is to completely respect the vulnerability and needs of these individuals, often without capacity. Vulnerability in another can be a very evocative experience and one certainly needs to be able to manage exposure on psychosis wards. A consultant psychiatrist brought to a ward group, a case of a homeless man who had been bludgeoned to death by a passerby whom he had asked for money, presumably due to the violence evoked by the vulnerability of the homeless man. Similarly, but on a much milder scale of reaction, I recall waiting in a very slow-moving post office queue in Waterloo once, whilst a middle-aged woman continuously and persistently verbally sounded off about a woman she had seen at the station, sitting on the floor and begging for money. On reflection, I considered that this woman was angry at the vulnerability exposure to the person begging on the street evoked in her.

With attention to the practical and emotional aspects of working with such vulnerable individuals in crisis, limits need to be set around: confidentiality, time and demand, especially when there may be 30 other patients on a ward, not all wanting help but some unable to ask for it or receive it. Individuals on the ward need help with grounding interventions and to help them to think about orienting themselves and about the sequence of events leading to their current admission to the ward or place of safety. This helps individuals gain a sense of past, present and future, which can appear to merge into one amidst confusions for a plethora of reasons, alongside the psychosis (substance use, non-medication use, lack of eating, bullying, domestic violence). It is alarming to see individuals who have been on the ward for many weeks still in an ungrounded, disoriented state, which can most frequently be dispelled fairly easily. I was aware with psychoanalytic training that I wanted to adopt an open-minded listening stance to these individuals to receive what they have to say and to consider what is being communicated at any time, rather than dismissing their communications.

I note that Herbert Rosenfeld held similar ideas about working with individuals with psychosis (Rosenfeld, 1988). I found that individuals initially need help to orient themselves and to be helped practically but therapeutically, for example, to the toilet, kitchen, nursing station or medication room. This holds very different boundaries to usual psychotherapy and is more in the realm of therapeutic support. For example, a person may be too afraid to go to the bathroom alone, due to past sexual abuses, especially when in an acute paranoid state. However, it is crucial to have understanding of the possible traumatic experiences brought to the scene of the ward and to show great sensitivity to individuals in this regard. Others, who were more settled in themselves, wanted to sit in a room one to one and to openly communicate about what was on their mind. Having worked with many individuals onwards, offering an empathic presence would significantly help, more so than I realised at first. I found that individuals were queuing up for a therapy space to talk about, for example, confusions, anger, upset, hurt at how family members have behaved, the police and their bruises, and so on. Invariably, the therapeutic space would take place in a quiet or family room on the ward. Nurses would advise as to who was suitable, regarding whether they posed a risk of violence to staff.

The usual boundaries of a therapy session regarding, for example, confidentiality and timing in private practice are different in the ward setting, and care needs to be taken in considering one-to-one work due to the risk of violence to self or accusations and complaints. Not one complaint was ever made about me in numerous years, and I think working carefully with patients and closely with the nursing and medical staff helped a lot with this. Firstly, I was offering one-to-one and group help to patients who would otherwise be bored, lonely or unhappy and gratitude was often felt by the patients for this, but not all the time. I witnessed a great deal of highly disturbed, acutely paranoid states of mind which was frankly unsettling in relation to the unpredictability of suddenly changing from one state of mind to another. Secondly, it was important to establish a positive and trusting relationship as quickly as possible, and I listened non-judgementally to what these people had to say and, therefore, helped them feel at ease and unafraid. I felt that the individuals on the wards were so eager to trust that they would easily become trusting once a consistent, genuine relationship had been established. I considered their attachment to me, encouraging independence and forming relationships with other staff and patients. Additionally, I thought about the transference to me from the group to the ward and was as careful as I could be regarding not evoking sibling rivalry.

The NHS mental health system is very hierarchical (power is from the top and instructions are to be followed, not questioned) and has a medication-based medical model structure. Therefore, it seemed that vulnerable patients are not necessarily cared for in terms of their emotional needs but are told what to do and when, hopefully with their best interests at heart but not always, as different priorities are made at different times and by staff differently trained. Nonetheless, the secure ward saves so many lives. Nurses are stretched with long shifts, low morale and pay, and being on the frontline for abuse and attacks from frustrated, angry, frightened and unwell individuals, it is not surprising that they may retreat to the nursing station. However, nurses' job is to be out on the ward ensuring safety at least. Current nursing training has started to include counselling skills, encouraging nurses to hold conversations with individuals on the ward. It's been a long time coming, perhaps indicative of the historically institutionalised environment of mental health hospitals eventually starting to dissipate. It's difficult to think about how individuals in mental health hospitals have been treated in the past and currently. We have histories of psychiatry which inform us of some of the horrific ways that unwell people have been treated and are treated like criminals. It has been unbearable for me to see how patients on the wards are left alone in rooms with persecutory hallucinations and delusions. I wanted to do something that may help in their recovery from crisis, so I went onto the wards, running groups and offering individual work to show some dignity and respect for these unfathomable states of mind.

I gladly, closely and supportively listened to hundreds of men and women on locked wards, each unique and moving, who told me their very troubling stories, and every time, I took what each said at face value, whilst reflecting on the meaning. I felt that a quiet, still presence was holding and grounding for these very vulnerable individuals. I would be clear about my role on the ward and the boundaries of confidentiality and note-taking. I didn't make any notes, and what each person managed to share with me was confidential apart from in the event of shared harm to self, other or from other. Often, I listened closely to very obscure narratives, and I admit not understanding all of it. It is profound to offer men and women a space to think about where they are and where they want to be and how to go about it, amidst internal and external disarray. In psychosis, it appears that the individual's inside is on the outside, with no protective 'skin' to contain this. I assessed material of a safeguarding nature, such as planned suicidality, safeguarding matters, including children, domestic violence and so on, contracting with individuals and gaining their consent to share such information with the nurses by way of handover, then entered electronically into the hospital notes. It is very important regarding dignity and transparency that individuals are aware when information that they share is then written into notes and accessible by other professionals on the electronic system and by the individual via a subject access request. The sensitivities and, therefore, potential for eruptions, especially with paranoia in the mix, lead to the need for great care to be taken in one-to-one work with these individuals. Facilitating safety is key through moment-by-moment observation of the processes of interaction – both verbal and non-verbal, conscious and unconscious. Establishing, developing and maintaining the therapeutic relationship is foundational, especially when misunderstandings and other ruptures occur. Consistency speaks to their inner anxieties of a sense of safety and security, when I observed them starting to relax. I was sticking by consistency for these individuals come what may, perhaps an experience of reliability for the first time in their lives.

Nurses would, at times, indicate which patients needed help and those who were not well enough for safe interaction. I followed up on every referral from the nurses and psychiatrists, offering one-to-one and group therapy to each. At times, nurses would enter the one-to-one therapy room with medication, and although this was their norm, for me, I needed to gently bring to their awareness that the patients needed to feel safe, without interruption, when sharing what was on their mind with me. This was a tricky dynamic since the nurses were in charge; however, having deliberately built a positive rapport with the nursing and medical team made these conversations easier. I was told that I should have put a 'Do not disturb' notice on the door, which I employed to help these individuals have some privacy and start to have a sense of safety for less than an hour. An interesting observation of one-to-one work with these individuals is that the boundaries of mind and body appear to me to be the core issue in relation to trying to clarify what is internal and what is external. When boundaries have been reputedly violated at a young age and in various ways, it is unsurprising that such confused minds are the result. Thomas Freeman et al. (1958), psychiatrists and psychoanalysts following Anna Freud, considered that the confusion for such individuals between their internal work and the environment at primitive levels, impacts important functions such as perception, thinking and memory. I think that this may be true at times, just as it is for those whose boundaries are, on the whole, intact. I have met individuals with psychosis whose assessments of people were consistently insightful and honest, where the medications caused cognitive decline. In many individuals, the anti-psychotic medications (e.g. Olanzapine) caused obesity due to the individual's brain telling them that they were constantly hungry, even after a meal. I agree with Freeman that the boundary between self and other is a central issue for this population, alongside issues of identity and attachment to their environment. Freeman observes this identity breakdown as substituting of the most primitive processes of 'merging with the object' for the typical adult forms of emotional relationship (Freeman et al., 1958). Offering consistent and reliable boundaries of time, setting, tone of voice and analytic stance with a friendly, kind yet if needed firm approach, had positive effects on helping individuals to feel more grounded and contained.

**Ward group work**

When first working on mixed psychiatric wards in London, group work was a natural progression when observing how individuals were isolated with very difficult psychic manifestations. I set up a meditation group, revealing just how agitated group members were, but many stuck with it and found some relief in participating. Another group I set up in London was an 'issues' group, where people could talk about what was on their mind, and this would cover, for example, anger and frustrations at the hospital system, the need for advocacy to appeal their section, complaints about nurses ignoring or violating them, violence from staff towards patients, complaints about the police, complaints about family members betraying their trust and calling an ambulance/police for hospital admission, claims about not being unwell, the food being poisoned and so on. I was able to manage groups well by first asking every individual on the ward, including nurses, regarding what kind of group would be helpful. I wrote all suggestions down, and each week, one suggestion would be the theme. Ground rules were suggested by the group and written on a flipchart.

I asked the group members to suggest types of refreshments to bring and bought these, being reimbursed through the ward petty cash. Managing the food needed thought, with all the feelings that food and family memories can evoke. However, I learned to manage this adequately through some lessons learned, for example, of individuals grabbing all the food at once. Other aspects of group work which needed thought were indicated when seeing patients one to one and in the group, due to the patient's transference onto me. However, on a ward, all patients are welcome to the group work held in the activity room. I discussed the possible emotional boundary difficulties with everyone I saw one to one and held absolute confidentiality. However, there would be transferential issues which could become potentially eruptive, such as when talking to someone else in the group after a one-to-one session with another in the group. I think that the issue was who was getting what from me, evoking historical thoughts and feelings, quite understandably; sibling rivalry is very powerful. All such matters were taken to psychoanalytic supervision and thought about in detail to keep everyone safe. I facilitated group work on the male and female acute psychiatric wards in London for many years, which was fascinating, enjoyable and of great value for understanding the inner recesses of the mind and how shared activity, such as arts and craft, can help engage a person to be able to speak more freely, share and feel less isolated and more empowered. I think that art group activity can really help individuals with busy minds to gain some respite and to focus on something visual.

# 2 Defining the psychoses and schizophrenias

'Madness in great ones must not unwatched go'.

*Hamlet*, William Shakespeare

Generally speaking, a person living with psychosis has 'imagined' views of their world of others, which may involve distortions arising from the person's particular issues. It may be considered that psychosis is generally due to intrusive factors: intrusive thoughts, a need for bodily/mind boundaries and differentiating between oneself and others – difficulties in distinguishing the individual's internal and external worlds, as further highlighted by Freeman et al. (1958). The psychiatrist Robin Murray has long been interested in uncovering the causes of psychosis to improve therapeutic options. Murray's work challenged the established perspective of schizophrenia as a brain disease with adult onset, instead showing that it is partly a neurodevelopmental disorder powered by insults to the brain during formative years (Dazzan et al., 2024).

This chapter intends to outline the psychiatric perspectives as laid out in the DSM-V (APA, 2013) on the schizophrenia spectrum, including psychosis, aligned with the descriptions of observations over many years on acute male and female psychiatric inpatient wards. Following depicting the psychiatric perspective, different views will be incorporated within the case studies, namely, the psychoanalytic perspective, as well as the systemic, cognitive-behavioural and humanistic schools in the form of discovering and processing different therapeutic approaches to helping individuals with psychosis. Demonstrating different therapeutic modality work with individuals living with psychosis intends to encourage all to strive to equip themselves to relieve the isolation of these individuals who I think are very much misunderstood and with whom many strengths lie. With firm kindness, curiosity and patience with oneself, along with good supervision, we can form a larger community of therapists who help individuals towards a better quality of life, at the same time improving our own quality of life by meeting such remarkable people and learning from what they teach us about our own minds and those of others. Additionally, as clinicians, we learn about the deeper realms

DOI: 10.4324/9781003509059-3

of the mind, with reference to better understanding the human condition. It is interesting to note that when asking people who have experienced psychosis if there is anything they would want different in their lives, every one of them have stated that they would not want to be rid of psychosis because of what it has taught them.

Individuals with symptoms of schizophrenia and psychosis, as seen in psychiatric settings, are often treated with eight to nine anti-psychotics, mood-stabilisers, anti-depressants and associated sedating medications to lessen the risk of harm to themselves or others or from others. These pills are designed to help the individual manage delusions, hallucinations, disorganised thinking, abnormal motor behaviour (including catatonia) and further negative symptoms. Anti-psychiatry may miss the extent to which individuals can become unwell and the risk this may pose to their own lives and those of others; however, there is a lot to be said for the convenience of medicating individuals often for life, without addressing the underlying conflicts and associated feelings. I consider the different medications filling in the gaps for what could have been given freely through better caregiving based on different transgenerational circumstances. Treatment of schizophrenia and psychosis in psychotherapy, with experienced clinicians, focuses on treating the disorganised, fragmented, unintegrated and fragile sense of self of the person. Psychotherapy would need to attend to nurturing an often severely neglected individual, who may not have experienced enough consistent and reliable caregiving and a holding or nurturing facilitative environment, where their locus of worth is internally focused rather than externally so. To add, insufficient parenting is often at no fault of the parents since looking back, their parenting is based on what they experienced and were exposed to both intergenerationally and transgenerationally. There are multiple possible external and internal varying circumstances, which input into parenting styles. However, adults do decide to have children, and responsibility needs to be taken to try to work through the hurts that might otherwise be passed on to their offspring. Often, this is the main difficulty: people being unaware of the impact of one's words and actions on others as caregivers, alongside the mechanisms of one's own mind and its impact on their offspring.

David Bell's perspective on paranoia is about managing internal anxiety: The threatening mental content is transported from its internal position and relocated in the external world . . . now objects in the external world appear to the individuals to be increasingly menacing, having been endowed with this 'projective significance', which, Bell considers, underpins mental states. Intolerable thoughts/impulses which cannot be acknowledged in consciousness become projected into figures in the external world. Individuals who are disposed to acute paranoid states of guarded suspiciousness can take on a delusionally convinced quality, becoming constructed into an elaborate delusional system of thinking (Bell, 2003). An example from my clinical experience is a patient who described seeing graffiti messages which he was totally convinced were about him, which set in train a paranoid matrix of distressing thoughts, taking the person to think his only escape was through a first-storey window, which he survived. A further example may be a woman's experience of being totally convinced that the television speech was referring to her, a belief which was immovable through therapy, despite her being able to understand the logic of my arguments about television companies recording programmes and not knowing her to refer to her.

Bell distinguishes between paranoid anxiety as universal and paranoia as a transitory state, whereby paranoid ideas can embellish a rationalisation for paranoid anxiety. The example Bell offers is that if one is convinced that others have sinister intentions towards them, there is justified reason to be anxious and be guarded (Bell, 2003). A further example of caregiving leading to great difficulties in the patient was a mother who offered 24/7 attention to her son, but this message needed to be decoded by him, since the reality was that she would demand 24/7 attention from him if the patient made themselves available by approaching the mother for assistance as she appeared to be offering. He lived in an understandably ongoing paranoid state of guardedness to the possible meaning underpinning his mother's utterances. His mother thought that the ATM machine knew that she didn't deserve any money. During the therapy, he felt that he was about to bump into another unstated rule like landmines. He had learnt to internalise his emotions, since his mother could not tolerate negative emotions expressed by him, wanting to uphold that her son had received a happy childhood, in stark contrast to her devastating childhood. This led him to hit himself in an attempt to take responsibility for how he felt and manage it, trapping him in a self-inflicting loop, which appeared sexualised. This loop was eventually extinguished in therapy when alcohol was dropped from his life and his anxiety was worked through in the transference.

Fortunately, as mental health is higher on the public agenda, which decreases stigma, more people are coming forward for therapy, increasing the likelihood of cycles of vulnerability being modified. Through my experience, vulnerability seems to be created by unexpressed anger; which the individual does not connect with for a plethora of reasons. It is striking and shocking, however, how many highly vulnerable individuals with schizophrenia and psychosis are turned away from numerous therapy services. One may wonder as to why so many therapists do not feel, able or willing to manage the risk or face the vulnerability perhaps of these individuals. Can you imagine what it is like for an individual trying to manage possible paranoid intrusive thoughts and persecutory audio and/or visual hallucinations, isolation, alongside medication side effects, then gaining the courage to start to think about sharing what is going on for them to another, only to be repeatedly told, 'Sorry, no one in this clinic can help you'? This is a very painful and regrettable situation, and it needs to change. Surely, more individuals and therapists need to better inform and equip themselves to help those diagnosed with schizophrenia or psychosis. Stating the risk excuse is unrealistic with this population, especially once a working alliance has been formed. In my opinion, we all need to show much more of an interest in our fellow human beings and educate and equip ourselves to be able to help those most in need, establishing and maintaining a sense of community, where we are much bolder and where members help each other reciprocally and willingly, rather than fearing difference, which can so easily turn into inappropriate and damaging hostility and resentment.

Many are as equally interested in the human mind as I am, and the benefits of individuals showing interest in some of the most vulnerable and isolated individuals is intrinsically life-giving, alongside being self-fulfilling and invaluable learning experiences both personally and professionally. The gratitude shown to me for taking the time to say hello to someone on a ward shows me how these people are used to feeling ignored and unworthy. It has become normal to ignore psychosis, as if it doesn't exist. There is furthermore an understandable unconscious or conscious fear of unimaginable states of mind. Let us now turn to consider other perspectives offering understanding of schizophrenia and psychosis in what follows.

There has been historical interest in psychosis from members of the psychoanalytic community since Freud, perhaps seeking to uncover meaning in the communications of individuals diagnosed with psychosis. Freud, however, paid more attention in his writings to neurosis rather than psychosis, which is interesting to consider in itself. Psychoanalytic thinkers have contributed hugely to unravelling psychotic processes, in my opinion. It may be worthwhile to examine some of the key figures who have shown such an interest in this population, starting with Eugen Bleuler. Doctor Eugen Bleuler (b. 1857–d. 1939) was born and raised in Zollikon, a village near Zurich in Switzerland. Following his graduation in medicine, he commenced his residential psychiatry training at the Waldau Hospital in Bern. For study trips, Bleuler travelled to Paris to work with Jean-Martin Charcot and to Munich, where he trained under Bernhard von Gudden, and also to London. Bleuler completed his residential training at the University Hospital of Psychiatry in Zurich, known as Burghölzli, and then was appointed director of the mental asylum of Rheinau in 1886. After living with and treating his long-term psychiatric patients in Rheinau for more than 12 years, he returned to Zurich as professor of psychiatry at Burghölzli in 1898 and held this position until his retirement in 1927. Eugen Bleuler died in Zollikon in 1939.

The term 'schizophrenia' was coined by Bleuler in the early 20th century. Bleuler considered that the symptoms of the schizophrenia condition, which include delusions, hallucinations, and disordered thinking, were the consequence of a split in the mind of the affected individual. Prior to Bleuler's work, this condition was referred to as 'dementia praecox', which means 'early dementia', and was considered to be a form of irreversible mental decline. Bleuler's book, published in 1911, focused on the history of schizophrenia research. Titled *Dementia Praecox or the Group of Schizophrenias*, it helped establish the contemporary understanding of schizophrenia as a disorder rather than a form of dementia and acknowledged the spectrum of schizophrenias. Today, schizophrenia is recognised as a chronic and severe mental illness affecting millions of people worldwide. How true is this? This book will attempt to more readily illuminate what constitutes the human condition in schizophrenia and psychosis. The story continues to consider what we can do to help individuals experiencing tormenting and dangerous symptoms to feel safer amongst us.

Initiated by the rejection of Kraepelin's main principle of nosology, namely, prognosis, Bleuler's belief in the clinical coherence of what Kraepelin had described as dementia praecox required Bleuler to seek different characterising features which would allow scientific description and classification. This led Bleuler to consider psychological and, to some extent, social factors, alongside an underlying neurobiological disease process, as constitutive of what he then coined as schizophrenia; therefore, Bleuler was an early proponent of the biopsychosocial understanding of mental health. Reevaluating Bleuler's conception of schizophrenia in the context of his overall clinical and theoretical findings, his paper provides a critical overview of Bleuler's key nosological principles, linking his work with present-day debates about naturalism, essentialism and stigma.

Whilst today, Bleuler is perhaps best known for the introduction of the term and concept of schizophrenia, or more precisely, 'the group of schizophrenias', this paper considers his work on schizophrenia principally in terms of its relationship to long-standing and complex theoretical debates in psychiatric nosology. This concerns the very nature of mental illness, in particular, the relationships between nature and mind and the individual and society. Debates about how nature – i.e. the brain and body – are related to the mind were highly topical with regard to mental illness in Bleuler's time and remain so today (Stier et al., 2014, 2013) as nicely captured in Lipowski's interrogative: 'Psychiatry: mindless or brainless, both or neither?' (Lipowski, 1989). Bleuler would have sided neither with a mindless nor with a brainless psychiatry but would have acknowledged both brain and mind, as well as social factors, as equally important elements in mental health and illness. He can thus be considered an early proponent of a biopsychosocial model in psychiatry.

There are varying diagnostic references used regarding the schizophrenia spectrum and other psychotic disorders, as discussed in DSM-V (American Psychiatric Association, 2013). However, although the DSM-V statistical manual can be considered a remarkable collection of observations by professionals, the DSM-V isn't the overruling influence in relation to how individuals with schizophrenia have been thought about and presented in this book. One may wonder about the degree of the medicalisation of human experiences and the linked diagnoses and medications, funding organisations. It may be helpful, perhaps, to start by clarifying what DSM-V states about diagnosing schizophrenia in what follows.

Psychosis is the umbrella term for a range of presentations, including those related to the schizophrenias (e.g. schizoaffective disorder, bipolar disorder) and psychoses (e.g. brief psychosis). Let us now turn to differentiate schizophrenia from psychosis, with the aim of providing an overview of these different diagnostic presentations, starting with some historical perspectives. It is, perhaps, noteworthy that it is more than a century ago since the depiction of *dementia praecox* by the German psychiatrist Emil Kraepelin. However, as stated earlier, the aetiology, pathophysiology and neuropathology in relation to schizophrenia remain ambiguous. Even though DSM-V (APA, 2013) and ICD-10, *Classification of Mental and Behavioural Disorders: Diagnostic criteria for research* (Geneva World Health Organization, 1993), provide criteria which encourage clinical reliability regarding diagnosis, schizophrenia, however, essentially appears to remain an ambiguous clinical syndrome explained by reported subjective experiences/symptoms, such as loss of functionality, for example, through behavioural impairments and varying patterns. Neuroscientific research purports various accepted biological markers linked with schizophrenia, including neurocognitive impairments, neurochemical abnormalities and brain dysmorphology. Medications for schizophrenia are known to cause cognitive dysfunction, therefore raising a pertinent query as to whether schizophrenia or the medication led to such impairments in cognition for this population.

However, none of these variables (DSM-V and ICD-10) have been definitively proven to possess sufficient sensitivity and specificity necessary of a valid diagnostic test. Genetic linkage and association studies have highlighted multiple candidate loci and genes but have failed to demonstrate that any specific gene variant, or any combination of genes, is either necessary or sufficient to be held as the cause of schizophrenia with any certainty. Therefore, the existence of a specific brain disease underlying schizophrenia remains hypothetical. In the context of ongoing increasing volumes of research data, the inconclusiveness of the search for causes of the disorder fuels doubts about the validity of the schizophrenia construct as presently defined. Given the mutability of the symptoms of schizophrenia and the poor coherence of the clinical and biological findings, such doubts are not without reason. It is interesting to consider what would be gained from pursuing a genetic cause of schizophrenia, potentially diminishing the role of parenting, and social and emotional factors in relation to the sense of self in schizophrenia.

Equally, it can be conceived that dismantling the concept of schizophrenia is unlikely to provide an alternative model accounting for the host of clinical phenomena and research data consistent with a disease hypothesis of schizophrenia. It seems that current opinion considers the clinical concept of schizophrenia as supported by empirical evidence in that its multifaceted format resembles a broad syndrome. It is evident that the diagnostic criteria of schizophrenia need to incorporate a trauma-informed perspective, likely resulting in most individuals diagnosed with schizophrenia being re-diagnosed with PTSD.

Turning to a summary of the different diagnoses within the spectrum of the schizophrenias and psychoses, DSM-V (APA, 2013) includes schizophrenia, other psychotic disorders and schizotypal (personality) disorder. These presentations are identified by abnormalities in at least one of the following realms, namely, delusions, hallucinations, disorganised thinking (speech), grossly disorganised or abnormal motor behaviour (including catatonia) and other negative symptoms. There are key features which define the psychotic disorders as outlined earlier and exemplified in what follows.

## Delusions

As defined in DSM-V (APA, 2013), delusions are beliefs held with such strong conviction that they become fixed and impervious to change via conflicting evidence. The content of delusional beliefs may include a range of themes, such as the following: persecutory, referential, somatic, religious or grandiose. *Persecutory delusions* are the most common beliefs, where the individual fears being harmed or harassed by an individual, organisation or other groups. *Referential delusions* are beliefs that particular gestures, comments or, for example, environmental cues are directed at oneself. *Grandiose delusions* occur when an individual believes that they have exceptional abilities, wealth or fame. *Erotomanic delusions* describe false beliefs that another person is in love with him or her. *Nihilistic delusions* are beliefs involving the conviction that a major disaster will occur. *Somatic delusions* are beliefs with a focus on preoccupations in relation to health and organ function.

It is clearly a sensitive area when assessing what is delusional, due to cultural and other variables. The criteria for assessing whether one's view of reality is delusional or not have been historically debated. However, according to DSM-V, a delusion is considered as such if it is deemed implausible and non-understandable to a peer from the same cultural background and if it does not derive from ordinary life experiences. An example of a 'bizarre' delusion is someone believing that a doctor in Germany has placed an electronic chip in their tooth through which the doctor is communicating with the individual. Delusions communicating a loss of control of mind and/or body are considered bizarre by DSM-V. Bizarre convictions include believing that one's thoughts have been removed by an external force (thought withdrawal) or that alien thoughts have been inserted into one's mind (thought insertion) or that the individual's body or actions are being acted on or manipulated by an external force (*delusions of control*). A non-bizarre belief is one where the individual is under surveillance by the police, with little convincing evidence. DSM-V states that it is, at times, difficult to differentiate between a delusion and a strongly held belief and it depends partly on the extent of the conviction with which the belief is held, in the context of clear or reasonable contradictory evidence in relation to the veracity of the belief. However, all of the above become more understandable when focusing on the emotional responses of these individuals. Now let us turn to consider hallucinations within schizophrenia.

## Hallucinations

Hallucinations are perceptual experiences, occurring without an external stimulus, as stated in DSM-V. Such experiences can appear clear and vivid as if normal experiences but are not under voluntary control. Hallucinations may present in any sensory modality (visual, olfactory [smell], tactile, gustatory or a general somatic hallucination). However, the most common in schizophrenia and associated disorders are auditory hallucinations. Auditory hallucinations are experienced as hearing voices, recognised as distinct from the individual's own thoughts. Not stated in the DSM-V is that auditory hallucinations can also be described by the individual as intrusive thoughts, usually not identified as their own thoughts. To meet the criteria for a hallucination regarding schizophrenia or a psychotic disorder, the hallucination would need to occur in the context of the parts of the brain or mind concerned with the reception and interpretation of sensory stimuli (sensorium). Hallucinations that occur whilst falling asleep (hypnagogic) or waking up (hypnogogic) are thought to be within the normal range of experience. Additionally, hallucinations may be an accepted part of religious experience in different cultural contexts. It seems further observable that differing sensory hallucinations are common during bereavement. Regarding religious experiences, a study was conducted in 2019 by Dudek, Krzystanek, Krysta and Gorna, entitled 'Evolution of religious topics in schizophrenia in 80 years period'.

The background of this study involved considerations that environment and culture are shown to be important factors influencing the characteristics of psychotic symptoms. The content of hallucinations and delusions is thought to be a projection of internal processes on the external world. Religion plays a central role in the lives of many people, but in schizophrenia, religious experience and spirituality is confounded by psychotic symptoms. The aim of this study was to find how the content of hallucinations and delusions interacts with cultural conditions that were changing over the decades. Regarding the subjects and methods: 100 case histories from 2012 were randomly selected. From the medical record, the content of hallucinations and delusions was extracted and categorised. Data from 2012 was compared with previous studies by the authors, obtaining perspectives on 80 years of history in the same hospital. The results demonstrate that religious content of delusions and hallucinations appeared in 26% of patients. Diversity of the religious and spiritual themes in schizophrenia has been gradually decreasing. Many minor religious entities and figures, such as saints and angels, disappeared in 2012. Although the occurrence of contact with God and other religious figures was similar to previous years, number of visions abruptly decreased. All of the religious content was culture-specific. Conclusions can be drawn in relation to religious topics expressing general plasticity over a time, following cultural changes in society (Dudek et al., 2019).

Now let us turn to consider disorganised thinking and speech, often referred to as 'thought disorder', which can be common on acute wards, especially when individuals are first admitted, mainly via a section, to psychiatric inpatient acute wards. Disorganised thinking can be recognised when an individual's utterances consist of incoherent groups of thoughts, which do not link together logically. There may be meaning to be discovered in such utterances, but at least it can be discerned that such individuals are very vulnerable when conveying this state of mind.

## Disorganised thinking and speech

An individual demonstrating disorganised thinking, or *formal thought disorder*, is recognisable from their format of speech. It can be inferred that an individual may typically jump rapidly from one topic to another, which is considered a phenomena of derailment or loose associations. Other signs of disorganised thinking are obliquely related or disconnected answers to questions (tangentiality). Speech can be, on occasion, so severely disorganised that it is incomprehensible, resembling *receptive aphasia* in relation to its linguistic disorganisation (incoherence). Since mildly disorganised speech is common and nonspecific, the symptom must be disorganised enough to substantially impair effective communication. The extent of the disorganised thinking may be difficult to assess due to a number of possible influencing factors, such as different linguistic background, substance use, traumatic experience and brain injury. Less severe disorganised thinking may occur during the prodromal and residual periods of schizophrenia. The prodromal period of schizophrenia includes nonspecific symptoms, such as lack of motivation, mood swings, social isolation, lack of concentration and sleeplessness. Such prodromal symptoms are not always easily observable, and diagnosis of schizophrenia can be, therefore, very difficult at this stage. The prodromal is the first stage of schizophrenia, followed by the active and residual stages.

Active schizophrenia involves recognizable psychotic symptoms as previously described, such as hallucinations and delusions. Individuals can require medical attention at this stage, depending on the content of the delusions and hallucinations, such as hearing voices instructing the individual to harm themselves or others. Clearly, a timely diagnosis and appropriate treatment can minimise the severity and frequency of distressing psychotic episodes. Interestingly, the residual stage of schizophrenia is no longer recognised as a diagnostic criterion, but it can help identify and monitor the progression of schizophrenia. In the residual stage of schizophrenia, hallucinations, delusions and disorganised thinking are mild or perhaps absent, although an individual may continue to experience symptoms from the prodromal stage.

**Disorganised motor behaviour (including catatonia)**

Grossly disorganised or abnormal motor behaviour may be demonstrated in a diversity of ways, ranging from hebephrenic childlike 'silliness', unpredictable agitation or puzzling sequences of behaviours. Difficulties may be observed in any form of goal-directed behaviour, leading to problems in performing activities of daily living.

Catatonic behaviour is a significant decrease in reactivity to the environment. Such behaviours range from resistance to instructions (negativism) to maintaining a rigid or bizarre posture to a complete lack of verbal and motor responses (mutism and stupor). Catatonic behaviour can include seemingly purposeless and excessive motor activity without obvious cause (catatonic excitement). Other features can be repetitive, stereotyped movements, such as staring, grimacing, mutism and echoing speech. Although catatonia has been associated historically with schizophrenia, catatonic symptoms are non-specific and may occur in other mental health presentations, such as bipolar or depressive disorders with catatonia, and in medical conditions, such as catatonia due to another medical condition. Let us turn to consider negative symptoms of schizophrenia and psychosis.

**Negative symptoms**

Negative symptoms account for a significant percentage of the morbidity linked with schizophrenia but are observed to be less prominent in other psychotic disorders. The two prominent negative symptoms in schizophrenia are diminished emotional expression and avolition. Diminished emotional expression includes reductions in the communication of emotions as observed in the face, eye contact, intonation of speech (prosody) and movements of the hand, head and face, which usually add emotional depth to speech. Avolition describes a decrease in motivated self-initiated purposeful activities. The individual may be observed sitting for long periods of time and show little interest in participating in work or social activities. Other negative symptoms include alogia, anhedonia and asociality. Alogia is manifested by diminished speech output, whilst anhedonia is the decreased ability to experience pleasure from positive stimuli or a degradation in the recall of pleasure previously experienced. Asociality refers to the apparent lack of interest in social interactions and may be associated with avolition or limited opportunities for social interactions. When diagnosing an individual, clinicians should firstly consider conditions that do not fulfil full criteria for a psychotic condition or are limited to one domain of illness. It is considered clinically appropriate to assess for time-limited conditions. Finally, the diagnosis of a schizophrenia spectrum condition requires the exclusion of another condition that may lead to psychosis.

## Psychosis

It is considered that psychotic disorders are from different origins, and the severity of symptoms can predict important aspects of the illness, such as the extent of cognitive or neurobiological deficits. The primary symptoms of psychosis are as follows: hallucinations, delusions, disorganised speech (except for substance/medication-induced psychosis), abnormal psychomotor behaviour and negative symptoms, as well as dimensional assessments of depression and mania. The extent of mood symptoms in psychosis has prognostic value and guides treatment. It appears that the schizophrenias and psychoses need redefining, particularly in relation to trauma-informed diagnosis and due to schizoaffective disorder increasingly being considered not a distinct nosological category. Many individuals with psychotic presentations demonstrate cognitive impairments in a range of domains, predicting functional status. Dimensional assessments of depression and mania in all psychotic disorders highlight mood instability for clinicians and the necessity for treatment where appropriate. Now let us turn to discuss the rather daunting-sounding schizotypal (personality) disorder.

## Schizotypal personality disorder

Schizotypal personality disorder is included within the schizophrenia spectrum and is included in a separate chapter of DSM-V (APA, 2013) named 'Personality Disorders' and similarly considered on the schizophrenia spectrum, also included in the European diagnostic guide in ICD-9 and ICD-10 (World Health Organization, 1977). The ICD-9-CM consists of the following: a tabular list containing a numerical list of the disease code numbers in tabular form; an alphabetical index to the disease entries; and a classification system for surgical, diagnostic and therapeutic procedures (alphabetic index and tabular list). The DSM is the diagnostic and statistical manual compiled and referred to in the USA.

The word 'condition' is being used rather than disorder since condition implies that the state of mind will change through medication, psychotherapeutic input, family and other support or a wide range of other factors, such as geography, socio-economic aspects and cultural and religious influences. A disorder can be considered as a state of confusion which would rarely be permanent, and therefore, the description of condition is preferred. The diagnosis of schizotypal personality condition describes a pervasive pattern of social and interpersonal difficulties, including reduced capability for close relationships, cognitive or perceptual distortions and eccentricities of behaviour. Such behaviours usually emerge in early adulthood but can also develop in childhood and adolescence. Unusual beliefs, thinking and perception are below the threshold in the schizotypal personality condition for the diagnosis of psychosis.

## Delusional disorder (DSM-V) (APA, 2013)

In order for an individual to be diagnosed with delusional disorder, the criteria are set out, such that there would need to be a presence of one (or more) delusions with a duration of one month or longer. Apart from the impact of the delusion(s) or its ramifications, functioning is not markedly impaired and the individual's behaviour is not considered bizarre or odd. It is interesting to reflect on how 'eccentric' behaviour is assessed as such or as disordered. Following many years of working on acute wards, it seems intuitive or informed by experience as to when a person's behaviour is eccentric or a manifestation of a disorder. If manic or major depressive episodes have occurred, these have been brief relative to the duration of the delusional period. The disturbance is not directly attributable to the physiological effects of a substance or another medical condition and is not better explained by another mental disorder, such as body dysphoric disorder or obsessive-compulsive disorder. Interestingly, Freud's initial statement about paranoia (Freud, 1896) remained markedly unaltered, namely, that paranoia involves the projection of intolerable ideas that are sexual. Freud distinguishes schizophrenic paranoia from obsessive-compulsive disorder, noting common features such as problems managing intolerable ideas, eventuating in self-loathing. Regarding obsessional neurosis, the intolerable idea is deleted through a repressive process, whereby self-loathing turns to self-distrust, and the obsessive individual then repeatedly checks and tries to correct their own utterances or actions, seemingly chasing an illusion of perfection. In contrast, for the paranoid individual, the idea holds, but the ensuing judgement is perceived as a threat from an external source (Bell, 2003).

There are at least seven subtypes to delusional disorder, according to DSM-V (APA, 2013). Erotomania applies when the central theme of the delusion is that another person is in love with them. The grandiose subtype is relevant when the central theme of the delusion is the condition of having some great but unacknowledged talent or insight or having made some important discovery. The jealous subtype applies when the central theme of the individual's delusion is that his or her spouse or lover is unfaithful. The persecutory subtype applies when the central theme of the delusion involves the individual's belief that s/he is being conspired against, cheated, spied on, followed, poisoned or drugged, maliciously maligned, harassed or obstructed in the pursuit of long-term goals. The somatic subtype is recognised when the theme of the delusion involves bodily functions or sensations. A mixed subtype is relevant when no one delusional theme predominates. The unspecified subtype applies when the dominant delusional belief cannot be clearly determined or is not described in the specific types, for example, referential delusions without a prominent persecutory or grandiose component.

Delusions are considered bizarre if they are clearly implausible, not understandable and not derived from ordinary life experiences, for example, an individual's belief that a stranger has removed his or her internal organs and replaced them with someone else's organs without leaving any wounds or scars. An individual's cultural and religious background must be taken into account when evaluating the possible presence of delusional disorder. The content of delusions is considered to vary across cultural contexts.

## Brief psychotic disorder

For this diagnosis to be valid, according to DSM V (APA, 2013), the following criteria need to be met (with the presence of 1, 2 and 3) 1. delusions; 2. hallucinations; 3. disorganised speech through, for example, frequent derailment or incoherence; and 4. grossly disorganised or catatonic behaviour. Additionally, the duration of an episode of the disturbance is at least one day but less than one month, with eventual full return to a premorbid level of functioning. Furthermore, the disturbance is not better explained by major depressive or bipolar disorder with psychotic features or another psychotic episode, such as schizophrenia or catatonia, and is not attributable to the physiological effects of a substance, such as a drug of abuse or medication, or another medical condition.

The essential features of a brief psychotic episode are the disturbance which involves the sudden onset of at least one of the following positive psychotic symptoms: delusions, hallucinations, disorganised speech and abnormal psychomotor behaviour, including catatonia. In addition to the five symptom domain areas identified in the diagnostic criteria stated earlier, an assessment also needs to be made of cognition, depression and mania symptoms, which are critical for differentiating between the various schizophrenia spectrum and other psychotic disorders.

## Schizophreniform disorder

According to DSM V (APA, 2013), the diagnostic criteria for this presentation need to include two or more symptoms for a significant portion of time during a one-month period (or less if successfully treated). At least one symptom needs to be 1, 2 or 3: 1. delusions; 2. hallucinations; 3. disorganised speech, such as frequent derailment or incoherence; 4. grossly disorganised or catatonic behaviour; and 5. negative symptoms, such as diminished emotional expression or avolition. The characteristic symptoms of schizophreniform disorder are identical to those of schizophrenia but is distinguished from schizophrenia by its difference in duration. The entire duration of schizophreniform, including prodromal, active and residual phases, is at least one month but less than six months. If the disturbance persists beyond six months, then the diagnosis should be changed to schizophrenia.

## Schizophrenia

Schizophrenia is diagnosed with the same symptoms as schizophreniform, with reference to DSM V (APA, 2013) as outlined previously, the difference being that in schizophrenia, the symptoms need to be present for a significant period of time during a one-month period of time since the onset of the disturbance or less if successfully treated. The symptoms need to interfere significantly with areas of the individual's life functioning, such as work, interpersonal relationships or self-care. Schizoaffective disorder, depressive or bipolar disorder with psychotic features and autism spectrum have been ruled out.

The characteristic features of schizophrenia incorporate a wide range of cognitive, behavioural and emotional dysfunctions and constitute a heterogenous clinical syndrome, impacting work and social functioning. Schizophrenia is recognised mainly through the presence of delusions, hallucinations and disorganised speech. Avolition involving a reduced drive to achieve goal-directed activity is associated with social dysfunction. A strong relationship has further been recognised between cognitive impairment and functional impairment in individuals diagnosed with schizophrenia.

There are cultural and socio-economic–related diagnostic factors in relation to schizophrenia, which need to be considered, especially when the individual and the clinician do not share the same cultural and socio-economic background. For example, ideas which seem to be delusional in one culture (for example, witchcraft) may be commonly held in another. In some cultures, visual or auditory hallucinations with religious content, for example, hearing God's voice, are deemed a normal feature of religious experience. Additionally, the assessment of disorganised speech may be difficult by linguistic variations in narrative styles across cultures. Furthermore, the assessment of affect requires sensitivity to differences in styles of emotional expression, eye contact and body language which vary across cultures. If the assessment is conducted in a language that differs from the individual's first language, caution needs to be exercised that alogia (poverty of speech) is not related to linguistic barriers. In specific cultures, for example, distress may take the form of hallucinations or pseudo-hallucinations and overvalued ideas which may clinically present as similar to true psychosis but are normative in the individual's subgroup.

The general incidence of schizophrenia tends to be less in females than in males, where the onset in females is at a later age, with a second midlife peak. Symptoms amongst females tend to be more affect-laden with more psychotic symptoms alongside an increased propensity for psychotic symptoms to women in later life. Women demonstrate fewer negative symptoms and less disorganisation. Social functioning tends to be more intact in females. According to DSM-V, approximately 5–6% of individuals diagnosed with schizophrenia die by suicide, whereas around 20% attempt suicide on more than one occasion. Suicidal behaviour tends to be in response to command hallucinations to harm oneself or another. Suicide risk remains high amongst males and females across the lifespan but more so for younger males with comorbid substance use. Other risk factors are depressive symptoms and hopelessness, being unemployed and following a psychotic episode or hospital discharge (APA, 2013).

## Schizoaffective disorder

The diagnostic criteria for schizoaffective disorder, according to DSM 5 (APA, 2013), are the following: an uninterrupted period of illness during which there is a major mood episode (depressive or manic), delusions or hallucinations for two or more weeks in the absence of a major mood episode during the lifetime duration of the illness. Additional symptoms include those that meet the criteria for a major mood episode and are present for the majority of the total duration of the active and residual phases of the illness. It would be important to disqualify that the disturbance is not caused by substance use. Schizoaffective disorder is more common amongst females, mainly due to an increased incidence of the depressive type among females.

## Catatonia

According to DSM V (APA, 2013), catatonia can occur in the context of several disorders, including neurodevelopmental, psychotic, bipolar, depressive disorders and other medical conditions. Catatonia is diagnosed in relation to the presence of three or more of 12 psychomotor factors. The main features of catatonia are the following: a psychomotor disturbance that may involve decreased motor activity, decreased engagement during interview or physical examination or excessive and peculiar motor activity. The clinical presentation of catatonia can be puzzling since the psychomotor disturbance may range from marked unresponsiveness to marked agitation. Motor immobility may be severe as in stupor or moderate as in catalepsy and waxy flexibility. Similarly, reduced engagement may be severe as in mutism or moderate as in negativism. Excessive and peculiar motor behaviour can be complex as seen in stereotypy or simple as in agitation, possibly including echolalia (involuntary repetition of another's words and sounds) and echopraxia (involuntary repetition of another's actions). During severe stages of catatonia, the individual may need careful supervision to avoid self-harm, harming others or harm from others. There are additionally potential risks from malnutrition, exhaustion, hyperpyrexia (exceptionally high fever) and self-inflicted injury.

In summary, the difference between schizophrenia and psychosis is that psychosis does not have the negative symptoms of schizophrenia but manifests all other diagnostic criteria, namely, delusions, hallucinations, disorganised speech and grossly disorganised or catatonic behaviour. Negative symptoms of schizophrenia can be recognised as lack of motivation, avolition, anhedonia, social withdrawal and emotional difficulties, such as alogia and affective flattening. These symptoms would clearly worsen the individual's quality of life.

# 3  Religious and spiritual considerations in relation to schizophrenia and psychosis

'The tempest in my mind. Doth from my senses take all feeling else.
Save what beats there. Filial ingratitude!'
*King Lear*, Act III, Scene IV – William Shakespeare

The majority of individuals, interestingly, whom I encountered on acute psychiatric wards, communicated via a religious lens. I have attempted to trace religious development back through the pre- and perinatal phases of life (Holmes, 2020) in an attempt to elucidate religiosity and forge possible links with mental health crisis – work which is ongoing in progress. It can be conveyed in different terms, namely, that hallucinations are experiences of perceptual force that occur in the absence of any actual external stimuli. Hallucinations are generally considered to be resistant to voluntary control. Whilst historically linked with mental disorder, they are currently considered to be more common amongst the general population than initially known. Hallucinations, not infrequently, portray spiritual and/or religious content and have been observed many times on acute male and female psychiatric wards, especially when individuals are in crisis or assessed as acutely mentally and therefore physically vulnerable. Spiritual experiences, including religious and mystical experiences, incorporate a wide range of experiences, amongst which are perceptual phenomena such as hallucinations, which can be of spiritual and/or religious significance. We might define spiritual experiences as those in some way involving a relationship with the transcendent. These experiences are necessarily subjective. We cannot know of them unless the individual experiencing them is willing and able to attempt to describe them. Both the experiences themselves, and any written or verbal account of them, necessarily involve interpretation. Experience is arguably not separable from interpretation. From the very time of having the experience onwards, prior assumptions about the world, including spiritual/religious assumptions, both shape the experience and become written into accounts of it.

Voices and visions, considered as part of spiritual experience, are encountered and documented in the sacred texts, hagiographies, biographies, autobiographies and other texts associated with most, if not all, of the world's

DOI: 10.4324/9781003509059-4

major faith traditions. Such experiences are of variable perceptual force and, at least in some cases, are not strictly hallucinatory. Even if they are, this does not necessarily invalidate the value and significance of the experience. It seems that the meaning of hallucinations needs to be rethought, without the overshadow of the diagnosis of severe mental health conditions, such as schizophrenia and psychosis. Voices and visions have been traditionally often understood as being, in some sense, 'revelatory'. Psychoanalysis has persisted to seek to understand the meanings of communications of those diagnosed with schizophrenia and psychosis, aiming to render such verbal and non-verbal communications as having meaning, rather than discarding them as nonsensical. Psychologists can find themselves hindered by individuals who are guided or instructed to, for example, pray, when it is clearly trauma or at least difficult or complex feelings that need to be processed. Finding a common ground is likely progressive, despite different uses of language referring to the same or similar-enough phenomena.

The concept of revelation generally includes some idea of communication with the Divine – whether directly or via some intermediary, such as a saint, angel or other spiritual entity. To qualify as revelatory, there appears to be usually the imparting of propositional information. Revelation may be public and thus shared with a faith community or else private and of significance only to the individual concerned. When spiritual experiences occur through voices and visions, revelatory experience has usually, historically, been considered in some way or another in terms of being 'supernatural' or miraculous. In the contemporary context, various other possible explanations for such experiences may be inferred, not requiring attribution to such mysterious forces. However, this does not necessarily negate their spiritual/religious significance.

We cannot know, scientifically speaking, exactly what the experiences of Moses were. However, the textual tradition is significant in its own right and is held to be authoritative. Whatever the actual experience of any historical Moses, the Abrahamic faiths have a sacred tradition of the communication of their God with human kind. In some sense or another, their God is said to 'speak' to his people, and they are said to hear his voice. This scriptural precedent for the expectation that their God speaks to his people – at least sometimes – paves the way for believers to have similar experiences. I will only take one such example here – from the Christian tradition – but there are countless others. Joan of Arc was born around 1412 and was burned at the stake in 1431, in fulfilment of the sentence passed by an ecclesiastical court convened by the English authorities in France. Her story is well-known, and there are good biographical accounts of her life, mostly based upon the evidence presented at the trials which led to her eventual death. Clearly, such accounts are not impartial – but they are also extensive and detailed. Joan's voices were interpreted at the time either as demonic or divine, according to one's interpretation. These views seem largely to have been politically determined. Much more recently, Joan has been canonised by the Roman Catholic church and, at the same time, has been diagnosed by various commentators as suffering from a psychiatric disorder. Her voices are thus ambiguous, although – whatever one makes of them – one can hardly fail to admire her courage of conviction in holding so faithfully to the truth of her experience despite such abysmal consequences.

Recent research, such as that conducted by Tanya Luhrmann (Luhrmann, 2012), Simon Dein (Dein & Littlewood, 2007; Dein & Cook, 2015) and others, has shown that in at least some churches, ordinary Christians today report hearing the voice of God out loud in response to their prayers. Such experiences seem to be not uncommon, albeit they are often infrequent in the lives of those who have them. They do not often seem to be like the experiences of Joan, and they do not always have perceptual force. However, they are significant for those who have them. What are we to make of such experiences? A reductionist scientific approach asserts that such experiences are invariably to be explained on natural grounds and that they are often (if not always) a manifestation of psychiatric disorder. Such explanations have been offered in respect of a wide range of biblical figures and saints, including the prophet Ezekiel, Paul of Tarsus, Joan of Arc, Teresa of Avila and even Jesus (taking some examples from the Christian tradition (Cook, 2012).

Everything is thus reduced to the domain of psychiatry, or at least neuroscience. At the other extreme, voices may be attributed to purely spiritual phenomena of a more or less miraculous kind. Generally, such attributions have been offered selectively, and there is a certain logic to the idea that one ought to be able to tell the difference between truly spiritual voices and those that arise from mental disorder, or at least there is a fine line to be drawn between the two. However, this view – which in the crudest cases amounts to a differential diagnosis between spiritual experience and mental disorder – is problematic. It involves making value judgements about other people's spiritual experiences, and it is not always completely clear what the basis for these judgements should be. In many cases, it seems to be assumed that in the absence of diagnosable mental disorder, the experience must have been a spiritual one. But why should this be the case? Can someone not be spiritually mistaken, or even downright wrong? Perhaps most importantly, however, the assumption seems to be that people suffering from mental disorder cannot have a spiritual experience.

This prejudice against mental illness seems both naive and stigmatising. If we just focus for a moment on auditory verbal experiences, why should their God only speak to people who are not mentally ill? Why should it not be the case that their God is more concerned about those who are mentally ill and thus more likely to speak to them? Perhaps mental illness confers a greater sensitivity to, and concern with, spiritual matters so that one might be listening more attentively. Of course, it will sometimes be quite clear that someone is ill and that their supposedly spiritual experiences are a product of their illness. However, this does not lead to dismissing such experiences as meaningless. At other times, it might be equally clear that someone is not ill and has had a positive and enriching spiritual experience. However, in many other cases, things are unclear and complicated. Wisdom is needed to discern what is going on. It may eventually be decided that a person is ill and that they have had an important spiritual experience. Or they may be diagnosed as ill and it may be unclear whether or not their spiritual experience is a positive one or not. It may take time to tell – and in some cases, spiritual struggles, which might be viewed as a good thing from one perspective and might still be viewed from another as having had a negative impact upon mental health and well-being.

The relationships between hallucinations, spiritual experiences, voices, visions and revelations are, therefore, not straightforward. Voices and visions may be of variable perceptual force and may or may not be strictly hallucinatory. Even if they are, this does not negate their spiritual significance, and checklists of criteria for making a differential diagnosis between spiritual experience and mental illness are often both stigmatising and naive. Reality is untidy and often ambiguous, not least in matters of mental health and spirituality. Discernment is clearly needed, and one can turn to Ignatius' teaching to learn more about this.

Religion and spirituality clearly play significant and influential roles within the lives of many individuals, including those with a diagnosis of schizophrenia. However, there is a paucity of information regarding the contribution of religion and spirituality to various domains of mental health, including, for example, the extent of mental health symptoms, explanatory models, seeking treatment, treatment compliance and outcomes. Let us look at the relationship of religion, spirituality and various domains in the lives of individuals with a diagnosis of schizophrenia or psychosis. Accessible evidence indicates that for some individuals, religion encourages hope, meaning and purpose, whereas for others, it evokes spiritual despair. Individuals with schizophrenia report religious hallucinations and delusions. Furthermore, evidence indicates that religion influences the extent of the symptoms. Religion and religious practices further affect social integration, suicide risks and substance abuse. Religion and spirituality further serve as an often effective means of coping with severe and enduring mental health experiences. Religion has been found to influence treatment compliance and outcome amongst individuals with a diagnosis of schizophrenia.

As discussed previously regarding the diagnostic criteria for schizophrenia and, more alarmingly, the individual's daily experience of delusions and hallucinations, schizophrenia is often a chronic, highly debilitating condition, as discussed previously, and is associated with impairments across multiple elements of functioning. The traditional psychiatric treatment of schizophrenia is based on the biopsychosocial model, often involving the prescription of anti-psychotic medications and psychological interventions in the form of talking therapies for the individual and accompanying family intervention. The biopsychosocial model of schizophrenia disregards the religious beliefs of the individual, although talking therapies and family interventions are very concerned with incorporating matters in relation to diversity, including cultural, religious and spiritual contexts. However, spirituality and religion have considerable influence in the lives of individuals with a diagnosis of schizophrenia and psychosis. This section aims to explore and evaluate the significance of the relationship of spirituality, religion, schizophrenia and psychosis.

To enable such an evaluation of the relationship between spirituality, religion, schizophrenia and psychosis, electronic searches were undergone using PubMed, Science Direct and Google Scholar. The search terms utilised were: schizophrenia, spirituality, religion, religious practices and religiosity. These terms were applied in differing combinations to identify the relevant articles, and articles which focused on a range of aspects of religion regarding schizophrenia were selected.

## Religiosity and religious practices among individuals with a diagnosis of schizophrenia

It is certainly interesting to consider the possibility of individuals with the psychoses and schizophrenias finding solace, belonging, recognition, attention, friendship and hope in religious communities and whether on balance this is a help or a hindrance. Homeless men and women are often provided with food via religious communities, and the most vulnerable in our society can gain shelter in religious buildings alongside a sense of connection with others. Research studies have evaluated different religious practices among individuals with a diagnosis of schizophrenia. For example, a Swiss study found that around one-third of individuals with a diagnosis of schizophrenia were very involved in religious communities. In the same study, a further 10% of the individuals were members of minority religious movements (Huguelet et al., 2006). A further Swiss study discovered that one-third of the individuals diagnosed with schizophrenia were very committed to their religious community, whereas another one-third felt that spirituality played a significant role in their life, carrying out daily spiritual practices, apart from involvement in a religious community (Mohr & Huguelet, 2004). International studies researching the religious practices of individuals with a diagnosis of schizophrenia or psychosis demonstrated that such findings are frequent in Europe (Kirov et al., 1998; Neeleman & Lewis, 1994) and in North America (Brewerton, 1994; Kroll & Sheehan, 1989). A further study discovered that 91% of diagnosed individuals reported being involved in private religious or spiritual activities, whilst 68% reported participation in public religious services or activities (Nolan et al., 2012). Further interesting studies, comparing religious practices in individuals diagnosed with schizophrenia and in the general population, indicate that religious involvement is higher among diagnosed individuals (Mohr et al., 2012), whereas others suggest that religious attendance is less in individuals diagnosed with schizophrenia (Cohen et al., 2010).

## Religion and mental health

Amongst the various aspects of religion and spirituality, the influence of religion and spirituality on human mental health has been one of the most explored areas of research. Generally speaking, delusions and hallucinations of religious nature are further categorised as those with religious and supernatural themes (Gearing et al., 2011). Religious delusions and hallucinations make direct reference to organised religious themes (e.g. prayer, sin, possession) or religious figures (e.g. God, Jesus, devil, Prophet). Supernatural delusions and hallucinations have more general mystic references (e.g. black magic, spirits, demons, being bewitched, mythical forces, ghosts, sorcery and voodoo) (Gearing et al., 2011). However, in the literature, delusions and hallucinations of either type are usually referred to as religious delusions.

Studies conducted among inpatients of schizophrenia indicate that the prevalence of religious delusions and hallucinations varies geographically, and the prevalence rates of the same vary from 6 to 63.3% (Krzystanek et al., 2012). Further studies, which have evaluated the delusional themes of various religious/spiritual delusions, report that common themes are those of persecution (by malevolent spiritual entities), influence (being controlled by spiritual entities) and self-significance (delusions of sin/guilt or grandiose delusions). Studies also suggest that when the non-content dimensions (conviction, pervasiveness, preoccupation, action, inaction and negative affect) of different types of delusions (persecutory, body/mind control, grandiose, thought broadcasting, religious, guilt, somatic, influence on others, jealousy and other) are compared, findings suggest that religious delusions are held with more conviction and pervasiveness than other delusions (Mohr et al., 2010). Data further conveys that diagnosed individuals with religious/spiritual delusions value religion as much as those without such delusions, but those presenting delusions with religious content report receiving less support from religious communities (Mohr et al., 2010).

Studies which have evaluated the religion in the context of psychopathology suggest that Christian patients have more religious delusions, especially delusions of guilt and sin, than their counterparts belonging to other religions (e.g. Islam). Other studies have shown that compared to Christians, Buddhists have a lower frequency of religious-themed delusions and that Protestants experience more religious delusions than Catholics and those without religious affiliations. Another study reported higher prevalence of religious delusions of guilt in schizophrenia patients of Roman Catholic affiliations, when compared to Protestants and Muslims. Cross-cultural studies which have compared people from different ethnic backgrounds suggest that in cases of paranoid delusions, Christian patients more often report persecutors to be supernatural beings, compared to Muslim and Buddhist patients. Other studies suggest that religious and supernatural themes in delusions are more common in Korean patients than Korean-Chinese patients or Chinese patients.

Greenberg and Brom (2001) investigated hallucinations of people belonging to Judaism and reported that hallucinations occurred more frequently during the night, linked to beliefs of the patients that they were more susceptible to evil spirits and demons at the night-time. Peters et al. (1999) compared patients belonging to Hinduism (Hare Krishna followers), Christianity and New Religious Movements with those of non-religious groups and found that patients from New Religious Movements scored higher on delusional measures than the other two groups. Other studies suggest that compared to the patients from Saudi Arabia, patients from the United Kingdom hear the religious-based auditory hallucinations more clearly (Kent & Wahass, 1996).

With regards to the relationship between religiosity and the presence of religious delusions and hallucinations, findings are contradictory with some studies suggesting higher prevalence of religious delusions and hallucinations in those with higher religiosity. It has been suggested that there is a relationship between religious delusions and cognitive impairments (Huang et al., 2011) and others suggesting lack of relationship between the two (Rudaleviciene et al., 2008).

Religious delusions have been found to influence help-seeking behaviour, treatment and outcomes. Evidence suggests that those with religious delusions take longer to establish service contact, receive more medications, have overall higher symptom scores and have poorer functioning (Siddle et al., 2002). Those with religious delusion/hallucination are more likely to receive magico-religious healing since they are often dissatisfied with psychiatric treatment (Huang et al., 2011) and are also more likely not to adhere to psychiatric treatment. Evidence also suggests that those with religious delusions have poor outcome and more frequently indulge in violence (Kraya & Patrick, 1997) and self-harm (Field & Waldfogel, 1995). There are some researchers who consider that religious delusions can influence health belief models and consequently lead to poor treatment compliance (Kelly et al., 1987).

In a review of 70 studies, the relationship between religion, supernatural beliefs and psychopathology were evaluated. Thirty out of the seventy studies (43%) have found a relationship between delusions and hallucinations and religion and the supernatural beliefs. The majority of the studies (27 of 30 studies) directly described religious delusions, of which 20 studies described delusions to be of a religion-based nature and 14 considered delusions to be of supernatural nature. Thirteen studies reported on religious hallucinations, with 11 having religious content and nine finding more supernatural content (Gearing et al., 2011).

Many studies have evaluated the influence of religion on the severity of psychopathology, and the findings tend to be contradictory. Some findings indicate that religious activities and beliefs are more frequently seen in persons who experience more severe symptoms, especially psychotic and general symptoms (Mohr et al., 2006), whereas others suggest that increased religious activity is associated with a reduced level of symptoms (Tepper et al., 2001). Data also supports that higher religiosity is associated with the absence of first-rank symptoms (Littlewood & Lipsedge, 1981).

### The relationship of religion and other clinical aspects in individuals diagnosed with schizophrenia

Researchers have discovered that religion/religiousness in individuals diagnosed with schizophrenia is linked with increased social integration, reduced risk of suicide attempts, reduced risk of substance use (Mohr et al., 2006; Huguelet et al., 2007), decreased rate of smoking (Borras et al., 2008), better quality of life (Cohen et al., 2010; Gaite et al., 2002; Murray-Swank et al., 2007), lower level of functioning (Huang et al., 2007) and improved prognoses (Flics & Herron, 1991). With regard to the relationship of religion and psychosocial adaptation, the findings are contradictory, with some reporting better psychosocial adaptation (Huguelet et al., 1997) and others reporting poor social and psychological status in a majority of patients (Mohr et al., 2012). Religious support and spirituality have also been found to be associated with better recovery (Huguelet et al., 2009; Webb et al., 2011; Mohr et al., 2007) and reduced relapse rate (Huguelet et al., 1997; Rund, 1990). However, in some patients, higher religiosity has been linked to higher risk of suicide attempts (Mohr et al., 2006).

## Religion and treatment adherence in schizophrenia

Various studies purport that religion/religiousness in individuals diagnosed with schizophrenia is associated with increased treatment adherence with psychiatric treatment (Kirov et al., 1998), whereas others suggest association of religion with poor treatment adherence (Borras et al., 2007). Other studies indicate that higher religiosity is associated with lower preference for psychiatric treatment.

## Religion and coping in schizophrenia

Religious coping can be multifaceted and refers to functionally oriented expressions of religion in times of stress. Religious coping is operationally defined as 'the use of religious beliefs or behaviours to facilitate problem-solving to prevent or alleviate the negative emotional consequences of stressful life circumstances' (Koenig, 1990). The concept of religious coping has been refined and categorised as helpful or positive, harmful or negative and with mixed implications. The positive religious coping strategies include religious purification/forgiveness, religious direction/conversion, religious helping, seeking support from clergy/members, collaborative religious coping, religious focus, active religious surrender, benevolent religious reappraisal, spiritual connection and marking religious boundaries. The negative religious coping strategies include spiritual discontent, demonic reappraisal, passive religious deferral, interpersonal religious discontent, reappraisal of their God's powers, punishing their God reappraisal and pleading for direct intercession (Pargament et al., 2000). The religious coping strategies with mixed implications include religious rituals in response to crisis, self-directing, deferring and pleading religious coping.

Few studies have evaluated the types of religious coping employed by individuals diagnosed with schizophrenia and their role in managing the stressful situation (Smith & Suto, 2012). Studies suggest that up to 80% of patients use religious coping as a means of dealing with their illness (Tepper et al., 2001).

Others have reported that in 45% of patients, spirituality and religiousness was helpful in coping with the illness (Mohr et al., 2010). Studies comparing different disorders suggest that patients with schizophrenia, bipolar disorder and schizoaffective disorder use religious coping for a significantly greater number of years and perceive the same to be more helpful than those diagnosed with depressive disorders (Reger & Rogers, 2002).

Some studies further suggest that religious coping influences other domains. For example, some studies imply that religious coping with individuals diagnosed with schizophrenia are associated positively with psychological and existential well-being, with positive religious coping being the primary predictor of psychological well-being (Pieper, 2004). A study revealed that benevolent religious reappraisal was associated with better well-being, better adjustment and lesser personal loss from mental illness, whereas punishing God reappraisal and reappraisal of God's powers were associated, with a greater correlation, with lesser well-being and adjustment and greater personal loss from mental illness (Phillips & Stein, 2007). Positive religious coping has further been associated with higher quality of life in the domain of psychological health, and negative religious coping has been associated with lower quality of life (Nolan et al., 2012) and higher distress, as assessed by the Depression Anxiety Stress Scale (Nurasikin et al., 2013). Longitudinal studies have shown that higher salience of religion and use of positive religious coping at the baseline are predictive of lesser negative symptoms, improved quality of life and better clinical global impression (Mohr et al., 2011). Participation in spiritual activities has been shown to be associated with better social functioning and dealing with negative symptoms (Revheim et al., 2010).

### Religion and explanatory models held by patients with schizophrenia

International studies have evaluated the explanatory models of illness held by individuals diagnosed with schizophrenia and suggest that many patients have non-medical explanations for their illness (Napo et al., 2012; Johnson et al., 2012). Most of the non-medical explanations across different studies pertain to the supernatural causes. The different explanations include obsession by witches or jinns (Napo et al., 2012), esoteric (Conrad et al., 2007), spiritual and mystical factors (Saravanan et al., 2007), family trouble, inner problems of self, economic difficulties, supernatural forces, sorcery, ghosts/evil spirit, spirit intrusion, divine wrath, planetary/astrological influences, dissatisfied or evil spirits and bad deeds of the past (Kate et al., 2012). A study from India reported that approximately 66–70% of the patients have at least one non-biomedical explanatory model of supernatural type (Kate et al., 2012), whereas studies from other parts of the world have reported the presence of supernatural explanatory models in about 10% of patients. A cross-cultural study which included Arab-Islamic, Jordanian and German patients suggests that Jordanian patients tend to believe more in esoteric factors underlying their illness, and they perceive the illness to be more threatening (Unal et al., 2007).

## Religion and quality of life for individuals with a diagnosis of schizophrenia

The World Health Organization (WHO) considers spirituality, religion and personal beliefs as an important area in the evaluation of the quality of life (QOL) (Culliford, 2002). The different mechanisms that have been proposed to link religiousness and spirituality to health outcome include behavioural (spirituality may be associated with a healthy lifestyle), social (religious groups provide supportive communities for their members), psychological (beliefs about God, ethics, human relationships, life and death) and physiological (religious practices elicit a relaxation response). Keeping the importance of religion and spirituality, the WHO designed a scale known as World Health Organization Quality of Life-Spirituality, Religiousness and Personal Beliefs scale (WHOQOL-SRPB). A study poses that spirituality and religiosity have an important influence on the overall QOL of patients with schizophrenia (Shah et al., 2011a). The same group of researchers further indicates a relationship between the spirituality and religiosity domains of QOL, as assessed by WHOQOL-SRPB, and the coping mechanisms used by the patients (Shah et al., 2011b).

## Religion and help-seeking behaviour

A study from India showed that many patients seek the help of faith healers to get rid of patient's symptoms (Kulhara et al., 2000), whilst it has further been demonstrated that indigenous healing methods are considered complementary to the medical management of mental illness (Saravanan et al., 2008). Interestingly, a survey of consecutive psychiatric patients attending a hospital in Tamil Nadu, South India, showed that 58% of psychotic patients saw a religious healer prior to psychiatric consultation (Compion & Bhugra, 1997). In fact, some of the studies suggest that seeking religious help for mental disorders is often the first step in the management of mental disorders, as a result of cultural explanations for the illness (Padmavati et al., 2005). Studies from other parts of the world suggest that patients with schizophrenia who are admitted for long durations experience spiritual distress (Yang et al., 2012). Studies which have specifically evaluated religiosity suggest that higher religiosity is associated with lower preference for psychiatric treatment (Huang et al., 2011).

## Conclusions and future direction

Despite the close relationship of religion with various aspects of schizophrenia, this area has been mostly ignored in mental health assessment, diagnoses and treatment (Brewerton, 1994). The limited existing data show that religion may have an influence on the expression of treatment-seeking behaviour, as well as treatment outcome. Given the importance of religion and spirituality for many patients, the biopsychosocial model of schizophrenia should integrate the same in order to achieve a whole-person approach to treatment. Findings also suggest that clinicians are rarely aware of the importance of religiosity for patients, even if spirituality needs are to be integrated into patient care. Hence, there is an urgent need to inform clinicians of this need of the patients, and to evaluate the religious and spiritual issues of their patients. There is a need to further evaluate this area, especially from cross-cultural perspectives. It is hoped that understanding the relationship of religion with various aspects of schizophrenia will lead to a better understanding of the patients by the clinicians, better organisation of services as per the needs of the individuals diagnosed with schizophrenia and better outcomes for the individual.

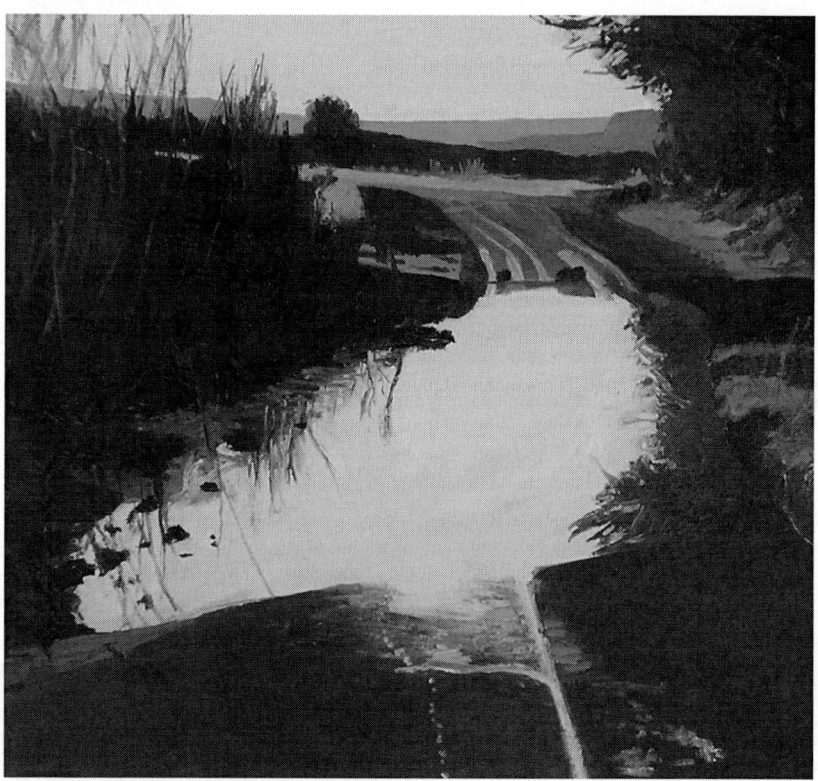

*Figure 3.1* Reflection painting

# 4 Organisational dynamics on acute psychiatric wards

'O, that way madness lies; let me shun that'.
*King Lear*, Act III, Scene IV, Line 21 – William Shakespeare

The UK mental health system is often referred to as the 'brick mother'. The National Health Service (NHS) was launched by the then Minister of Health in Attlee's post-war government, Aneurin Bevan, at the Park Hospital in Manchester. The motivation to provide a good, strong and reliable healthcare to all was finally taking its first tentative steps. At its founding in 1948, it was guided by three core principles: that it provides to the whole population (universality), that it be free at the point of delivery and that it be based on clinical need, not ability of pay (equity). The UK mental health system structure is very hierarchical, and therefore, power stems from the top down, meaning that staff appear to be expected to do as they are told and not to challenge authority. Many staff stay in the role for many years, mostly secure in their positions, especially as groups of colleagues inevitably form over time, supporting or covering one another, which, of course, can become unhealthy. New blood in the form of new staff, coming in with fresh eyes, is often considered a threat, and the invaluable information that new minds bring to the work situation often appears unwelcome, inviting threats from the established staff group, including bullying and unfair dismissals. If there were well-trained, confident groups of staff on wards or units, then they would welcome new feedback, and this could input into innovative and more effectively run units, which would inevitably be safer for both patients and staff. Some of the incidents in the mental health system are very unsafe and at time fatal, placing staff and patients at risk, in an environment where health, safety and safeguarding are supposed to be prioritised.

For example, a staff member reported having been new in post but not having been instructed on basic safety information. I reflected on the seemingly shut-down nature of the staff responsible for such neglect, not able to feel concern – presumably having worked exposed to trauma for too long and unable to feel any longer, acting dangerously without awareness or care, whilst nobody appeared to notice, amongst similarly emotionally shut-down

DOI: 10.4324/9781003509059-5

staff, viewing especially patients on long waiting lists like annoying pests to be ejected (patient safety issues). Another staff member recounted seeing a patient in therapy who had experienced three previous sudden endings, when the therapist had, for one reason or another, left with no explanation, leading to the patient attempting suicide, presumably due to repeated abandonments. How was this allowed to happen for a fourth time? There is presumably something being enacted by supervisors who can't/won't take proper notice of the likelihood of such repetitions or perhaps sadistically enjoy such pain caused in another.

The following musings reflect a lifetime's professional experience of working with individuals on acute, assessment, crisis and rehabilitation wards with individuals in profound crisis, working through life and death issues. Thankfully, those on these wards have survived and are safe, in that they have professionals around them monitoring their movements and access to objects and substances. The secure ward is both needed, rejected and reviled by those who are so acutely ambivalent about wanting to live or die. It seems fair to state that many living through psychosis are not at times aware of their vulnerability and the risky consequences of their decisions, possibly influenced by voices instructing them to kill themselves or others, the responsibility for which is passed to the mental health team.

For over 17 years, alongside individual work, I set up and facilitated activity groups on both male and female wards and in the hospital place of safety (a small mixed ward with six to seven beds for men and women usually detained and sectioned by the police, posing an immediate risk to themselves and/or others/from others). It was possible, on occasion, to hold a conversation with a few patients in this environment, but most of the time, it was too dangerous to even enter the ward due to the acuity of the disturbance and risk of violence to staff. I felt suffocated at these times in my countertransference, perhaps indicating the trapped nature of these very acutely unwell individuals. The occupational therapist stayed for four months but could not develop her work, complaining about the team dynamics and ward politics as reasons for her departure. It seems frequent that when working on inpatient and outpatient units that it is less difficult working with the patients than the staff. This may, in my opinion, be about management not wanting to take responsibility for their shortfalls and this being blamed on nurses who become resentful and demotivated. Another reason may be the extent of trauma that the team are trying to manage, possibly causing splits in the team, leading to conflict, polarisation and animosity.

Patients are moved usually within a few days from the place of safety to one of the hospital acute wards or a psychiatric intensive care unit (PICU). The PICU houses patients in separate male and female units, who find it more difficult to manage their state of mind, often resulting in violence. It was helpful to have talked with patients in the place of safety, who, after around 48 hours, had either sobered up or recovered enough from substances or a very acute but brief psychosis, to gain insight about how they came to be in this difficult space. The place of safety, like most acute wards, are not places one would want to return to.

Patients shared with me about how frightened or terrified they were, leading to violence against perceived threats from the public or family and then to police intervention, which could be helpful but, at times, was not. Individuals may be involved with sex work and substance addiction, alongside mental health vulnerabilities. The staff were often the only source of care for some individuals, such as a sex worker who unfortunately was addicted to crack cocaine and had a history of psychosis. Despite having a flat, her voices told her to live on the street, where it seemed she was addicted to having sex, believing she 'had to have sex daily', doing so for money in exchange for crack cocaine. Having become pregnant, she was found on the streets barefoot, wandering into charity shops and sleeping outside food stores. She was very underweight, gaunt and expressionless with old food in her highly matted hair. Undergoing therapy on wards requires tolerance of extreme vulnerability. It took several months for this young woman to accept that she was pregnant, and when she could manage a back-and-forth conversation after several months on the ward, she was able to share her family contact details. When the father and sister were contacted regarding the possibility of her returning to her home country, the response was that they wanted her to stay in the UK. The extent of her abandonment was stark. She literally had no family to turn to, which was gutting in my countertransference. The shame of the team knowing that her family didn't want her caused further violent eruptions from her. The team were able to hold this deeply painful situation, just about.

Another similarly aged, early thirties female was brought to the acute ward, with highly matted hair, underweight and silent. She had been found outside a food store, begging for money whilst seated on the street with no underwear on and a very short skirt. Passers-by had reported this to the police, and due to her lack of mental capacity, they had sectioned her into a secure hospital setting. The young woman was similarly very streetwise and addicted to crack cocaine and heroin, and when she absconded from the ward, social workers found her lying in bed surrounded by drug paraphernalia and her door open to anyone walking in and out. This young woman was controlled by a group of drug dealers and was unable to protect herself. This young woman fascinated me, and I realised that I was being seduced by her, as she knew well what to do in sex work around a crack cocaine addiction. I wondered what she wanted from me and discovered through her non-verbal communications that it was food, which I fetched for her. I consider what other kind of nurturing they are perhaps seeking too. Becoming close to individuals in acute psychiatric wards takes great care and caution due to the often sudden shifts in moods and states of mind.

When leading on groups, all of which were risk assessed and stemmed from what the patients wanted, it was most difficult to organise groups on the male ward, which I have reflected upon. The atmosphere on the male-only acute wards was often very violent, with acutely unwell men involved in substance misuse, street homelessness, neglect, refugee or asylum-seeking status, sex work, HIV-positive status or forensic backgrounds. Often, patients needed to be deported or returned to their home country, much against their will. These patients were escorted by two burly nurses on the plane back to their home country. Over time, the male patients became more familiar with me, as I with them and the ward culture. Being female on an all-male ward had pros and cons but remaining calm was key, even in the face of some extremely frightening and potentially extremely dangerous situations.

I think that the mental health systems are inevitably very painful places to work. Many staff are unmonitored in the wider hospital context, perhaps unmotivated by low pay or lack of recognition. It is interesting to have observed how the person who speaks up about safeguarding concerns becomes ostracised, as if the person speaking up about safety matters has done something wrong. Ward dynamics seemed healthier with a largely convivial and diverse team of ward staff who were able to laugh appropriately to manage the situations at hand and maintain a team spirit. What was most noticeable was that some senior staff behaved atrociously for self-gain, presumably consciously and unashamedly (for example, writing clinical notes under someone else's name to avoid responsibility or avoiding doing their job, then blaming the newest or youngest staff member with a coterie of colleagues to support them with their blaming). This can be a dangerous environment, where right and wrong have lost their meaning and one is expected to endure one abuse of human rights after another.

It perplexed me as to why individuals placed themselves on a three-year waiting list for treatment, which they could gain from free alternatives easily sought online or via their GP. Triage assessments were carried out for those on the waiting list, and many had been waiting for three years for treatment in psychotherapy. I helped individuals become aware of other alternatives, such as therapy in training organisations, where low-fee therapy would be offered but supervised by much more experienced practitioners, of which there are many (although reducing) in London and other UK locations. There is also a plethora of free and low-fee counselling options, in-therapy training organisations, online resources and therapists who offer a sliding scale of fees. I am still pondering about the possible masochism involved in staying on a waiting list. Perhaps there is some perceived safety in remaining on a waiting list offering, for example, potential hope, recognition, belonging, identity and purpose. Such waiting lists need to be carefully managed in relation to risk. It was perplexing to me how waiting lists accumulated, with little constructive effort invested in reducing them through a structured process of a certain number of sessions for each individual, which at least would give a foundation to be built on in further self-care. Instead, various manipulative methods were used to reduce the list of patients waiting by some seemingly sadistic managers, which was wholly unacceptable. Reporting such crimes fell on deaf ears since there appeared a common deafness where reporting ran the risk of further marginalisation for acting ethically or threatened by constructive dismissal. If you are prepared to turn a blind eye to harm being caused and keep stum, you will stay and at least have an income. However, the cost to one's integrity and, therefore, conscience and quality of sleep is high for those whose consciences are intact. The perhaps compelling attraction to collude is acceptance into a club of staff who can and do deceitfully cover for each other. This dynamic creeps into accrediting organisations, whose reputations are saved by practitioners covering for each other; another layer of collusion regarding the fib of practitioner monitoring and patient safety is very concerning. In the vein of understanding organisational dynamics regulators, appear mostly comprised of administrators, who can appear unconcerned about some of their members apart from their membership fee, who, like the waiting list patients, become numbers, no longer considered as humans. Let us now turn to consider different perspectives regarding the asylum.

## A note about Henri Rey

John Steiner is a psychiatrist and psychoanalyst, who worked at Maudsley Hospital for many years. Steiner wrote about Henri Rey with fondness, while Rey wrote about his experiences at Maudsley Hospital, where he, too, worked, with a similar quality of fondness. The psychoanalytic method seems to attract contention, perhaps reflecting the very conflicts which it seeks to observe, think about and try to resolve. Dr. Henri Rey was born in 1912 on the island of Mauritius and was of French ancestry. By all accounts, Rey profoundly influenced generations of new psychiatrists and psychoanalysts training under him during his 32 years at the Maudsley Hospital.

Steiner considered that although Rey was in some ways an anomaly in an institution which was frequently hostile to psychoanalytic ideas, he considered Rey to have helped trainee psychiatrists to make sense of the confusing and disturbing phenomena which they encountered when working with borderline and psychotic patients. Through the application of psychoanalytical ideas, Rey encouraged and facilitated them to seek and find meaning in much that was otherwise incomprehensible. Steiner reports Rey having a special affection for the Maudsley, which he referred to as 'the brick mother', a phrase referred to earlier. He saw how important the secure hospital was, as a place of safety, for patients who were afraid of breaking down and for whom it offered continuity and stability. In 1977, Rey retired to the Ile de Ré in western France, where he led an active life until his death in 2000.

It seems that despite Rey's French ebullience, Rey was a shy man, not giving a paper in the psychoanalytic society until he had retired. He was nevertheless greatly influenced by his analysis with Herbert Rosenfeld and his supervision with Joan Riviere. Rey's ideas are not so well-known, and Steiner states that he thinks that they should be better known. Rey's major work,

*Universals of Psychoanalysis in the Treatment of Psychotic and Borderline States,* was only published in 1994 (Rey, 1994) and seems to yet to be fully assimilated by psychiatrists and psychoanalysts. Rey's main tenets of the mind are outlined later and hope to be of some interest to readers.

## A model of the mind based on spatiality

Pivotal to *Universals of Psychoanalysis,* and to Rey's main approach to patients, is his acknowledgement of conceptualising the mind in relation to spatial terms. Rey described how often patients feel prematurely pushed out of the maternal space (inpatient holding ward) before they are ready to face the exposures of life. Often, an intermediate space emerges within the mother's care, conceived by Rey as the 'marsupial space' functioning similarly to the pouch of a kangaroo, offering access to the external world alongside the safety and familiarity of the mother's protection.

Many patients who are very unsettled and disturbed for many reasons, find it difficult to find an area of safety: where they easily feel that they are too close to their objects (other people) and feel trapped and unfortunately develop a claustrophobic reaction; when they try to escape, they feel agoraphobic, terrified of empty and undefined spaces which threaten them with a frightening sense of disintegration. Rey managed to formulate this observation in terms of what he then called a 'claustro-agora-phobic dilemma', where the patient is able to find safety and security neither with objects nor away from them.

## Borderline phenomena

Rey was particularly interested in and developed a deep understanding of individuals with borderline states. He understood this interesting term not only to designate a diagnostic group of patients but also standing as a metaphor describing the way in which such patients unconsciously develop the structure of their mental space and the position they occupy within it in relation to the way that their parenting has been demonstrated. Additionally, Rey recognised how borderline patients find choices so difficult to experience, such that they choose an area between two alternatives, in particular, when issues of identity are involved. The borderline patient feels s/he is neither fully male nor female, neither large nor small, neither inside nor outside but on the border between these myriad states, which is extremely difficult for them and those around them.

## Endo and exo-skeletons

Rey made a distinction between internal and external sources of identity. Agoraphobic states of mind lead to seeking an object (relationship) within which to reside and attempt to experience safety, which Rey describes as an exo-skeleton. In this case, similar to a crab or mollusc, the individual surrounds himself with an external structure, but such safety, of course, depends on the continued availability of the external object (relationship). Rey considered that genuine security requires an internalisation of structure, creating an endo-skeleton, or backbone. For the endo-skeleton to develop, the individual needs to find the confidence to emerge from the maternal space and approach the object from a position of separateness to enable being able to take something in and, from this, create an endo-skeleton.

## Reparation

It is considered that Rey's paper on reparation is a classic, describing how central this concept is, as described earlier, for the working through of loss and despair. With the realisation of the importance of symbolic function, Rey addressed the difficulties that face an individual who is unable to symbolise properly. Rey was struck by the impossibility for such individuals to make reparation, and although the emphasis is on the individual patient's state of mind, this can only be fully understood by considering how such an individual is responding to the behaviours and communications of the caregiver/s. Additionally, Rey posed that due to the prevalence of concrete thinking amongst such individuals, the damage that they have caused to their internal objects is experienced as real and actual, and as a result, the repair which the damaged object demands is equally real and actual. This can best be understood in relation to different parts of the personality structure of the individual. From Rey's perspective, such concrete repair is largely beyond the means and resources of any individual, and he demonstrates how this is one of the factors encouraging emerging states of omnipotence alongside a shift towards manic pseudo-reparation. This understanding of such failures in reparation motivated Rey to closely observe what it was that his individual patients specifically wanted or needed from their treatment. Rey discovered that it was often the repair of an object which they had damaged, or felt they had damaged, which was the primary purpose for their analysis. Once the object had been dealt with, they then feel that they were able to ask for anything for themselves and, therefore, start to meet their own needs.

## Symbolic function

Henri Rey was particularly concerned with the difficulty of how it is that a mental representation transforms from the concrete to the symbolic. Like many of his contemporaries, he emphasised the link to death, mourning and loss. It was thought by Rey that it is only as the object is relinquished and mourned that it can be internalised in a transformed state. To illuminate this process, he quoted by heart the beautiful poem *Le Cimitière Marin* by Paul Valery, illustrating transformation:

> *Comme le fruit se fond*
> *en jouissance*
> *Comme en delice il*
> *change son absence*
> *Dans une bouche où sa*
> *forme se meurt*

(As the fruit melts in the enjoyment, transforming its absence into delight within a mouth in which its form is dying.) John Steiner is to be thanked for summarising Henri Rey's contribution, and more information can be found on the Melanie Klein Trust website (Steiner, 2012).

## The psychotic wavelength

Another major contributor to helping understanding those working with individuals presenting with schizophrenia and psychosis in relation to organisational dynamics, is Richard Lucas who wrote *The Psychotic wavelength* in 2009. *The Psychotic Wavelength* offers a clinical psychoanalytical framework for use in everyday, general practice in psychiatric settings and discusses how psychoanalytic ideas can be of enormous value, when used to help seriously disturbed and disturbing psychiatric patients with psychoses, including both schizophrenia and the affective disorders. The linking of psychoses, schizophrenia and the affective disorders is extremely helpful in grasping the similarities, overlaps and differences between these seemingly separate diagnoses, as a practitioner. In his book, Lucas advocates that when clinicians seek out to help psychotic patients, the central concern should be to clarify what is happening during the process of their breakdown, which can be gleaned through close ongoing observation in their different situations, such as mealtimes, group work, communication or attitude towards medication, amongst many others. Lucas portrays this as tuning into the psychotic wavelength – a process allowing clinicians to differentiate between and address the psychotic and non-psychotic parts of the personality, which Bion refers to as being endemic in every human being (Bion, 1955). Bion considers that the distinguishing of the psychotic from the non-psychotic parts of the human personality relies on a minute splitting of all the parts of the personality concerned with awareness of internal and external reality and the expulsion of such fragments, such that they enter into or engulf other individuals pertinent to past relationships (objects). Many carers of family members who suffer the insanity with and for their loved ones, with the psychoses, schizophrenias and affective disorders, express disdain at Bion's representation of such severe mental health difficulties, through such everyday terminology as if psychosis is a mild phenomenon.

Men and women on acute wards diagnosed with psychosis, schizophrenia or affective disorders suffer enormously with highly anxious and paranoid episodes, frequently and daily for up to seven hours, often leading to persecutory and persistent voice-hearing, intrusive thoughts and instruction to harm their self or others or to take their own life or that of others, alongside being harmed by others. This extreme suffering, experienced on an everyday basis, coupled with an inadequate understanding of one's own condition and that of others, leading to social isolation, loneliness, unemployment, marginalisation, homelessness and a lack of opportunity, would naturally be of severe detriment to people with these conditions. Medication can adequately manage such states of mind in many cases, but the neglect which circles to self-neglect and lack of motivation through fear can be very debilitating. It is well-researched that individuals diagnosed with psychoses and schizophrenias live a higher quality of life when supported by their families. However, it is also researched that families especially with highly expressed emotion, is unhelpful perhaps for anyone but especially those with sensitive dispositions who have experienced adverse childhood experiences.

## The logic of emotion

Bion (1955) offers a revolutionary way of thinking about our own minds, shifting the concept of psychosis from being solely applicable to the external world and relevant only to others, to considering the dynamic 'in-house', so to speak, which is illuminating. From observations reflected on and reconsidered for over 15 years of working on acute wards with children, young people, men and women aged 8–65 years old, as Bion indicates, there is always, in my experience, a normal/ordinary aspect to the individual diagnosed with the psychoses and schizophrenias, with whom one can hold a back-and-forth conversation with. Many times, when working on acute wards, and listening to patients obsessively repeating the same sentences in great distress, intervening to ask, 'Would you like to have a conversation with me?' or 'What are you interested in?' always gains a straightforward response. It is interesting to wonder about why this ordinary aspect of the person becomes so buried or hidden in what appears as florid psychosis often. It is, therefore, worth considering what it is about the person that is driving them and those around them mad. I think that Bion and years of observation and engaging with men and women with the psychoses and schizophrenias, brings me to value the importance of rationalising what is occurring for each individual manifesting these conditions. For example, recognising that aggression often hides great fear, and therefore, speaking to the frightened part of the vulnerable person with empathy, can create a sense of safety and security for the person who, therefore, no longer needs to be aggressive. Therefore, there is a logic that needs to be considered and applied in such situations in order to properly help these extremely vulnerable individuals and families to feel that they can be with another. It is, perhaps, the process of applying logic to acute emotional states.

## Engaging with the ordinary in the psychoses and schizophrenias

Lucas further postulates that if clinicians can recognise the psychotic wavelength, then inevitably, they can assist the individual to come to accept the realities of living with a psychosis more effectively. However, I think that the ceiling needs to be raised. My observations lead me to think (I do not claim to be the first person to think in this way) that individuals with a diagnosis of psychosis and schizophrenia at base have a disorganised or chaotic or neglected sense of self, so much so that their minds have lost all sense of boundaries, especially observed in paranoia and OCD aspects of these conditions. If it is conceivable that a wavering sense of self underpins the psychoses and schizophrenias, then this can be treated in psychotherapy, as is practiced by this author, with regular supervision in place, as with all other clinical patient/client work. Of course, additional symptoms in individuals with a diagnosis of schizophrenia and psychosis need to be taken into consideration, and risk assessed. Professor Emeritus Robert Hinshelwood, who has studied and written about psychosis for many years, in fact encouraged and supervised my work with individuals and families with psychosis and schizophrenia for over seventeen years. He helpfully states in *Suffering Insanity* (Hinshelwood, 2009) about how Freud made observations in his famous Schreber case, where the patient was seen to converse later in his illness in ordinary ways in accordance with his role as an appeal court judge, whilst at the same time harbouring delusions and beliefs in his reconstructed world (Hinshelwood, 2009). Additionally, Freud's (1901) much overlooked text, indicates that a reality-seeking aspect of the mind of the individual with schizophrenia consistently survives through the extremely painful episodes of a psychotic nature, such that:

> One learns from patients after their recovery that at the time in some corner of heir mind (as they put it) there was a normal person hidden, who, like a detached spectator, watched the hubbub of illness go past him.
>
> (Freud, 1940, p. 202)

## Further notes on organisational dynamics on acute wards

The structure of psychiatric wards may be pertinent to help understand the context. Psychiatric wards have different levels of functioning, ranging in purpose from the assessment ward, which could be a place of safety, or acute ward, depending on the acuity and risk of disturbance, or where patients are brought or who present themselves voluntarily to be assessed and moved to the appropriate next step, to PICU, forensic and rehabilitation wards, or to supported accommodation as a move into the community, or a return to their home. There are a lot of returning patients to the wards, with a high percentage with dual diagnosis, including substance misuse, sadly, alongside other risky and self-harming behaviours. For example, all inpatients, if this is one way to describe the people on the ward, are there for their own safety. Many do not seem to be aware of this at the time of their crisis, a main reason for their safety needing to become statutory. It is understandable that a part of them can be very angry about being held against their will, when a Section 2 or 3 is imposed on them, under the Mental Health Act. In the Middle East, there is not a Mental Health Act, and mental illness is considered more akin to a crime, which can't be discussed outside or presumably within the family. In the ward groups, it can be surmised that feelings and thoughts are brought regarding their freedoms being curtailed and risk of harm, which perhaps helped contain very distressed individuals. It can be considered that the inpatient ward becomes the parent, certainly evoking childhood and adolescent responses and reactions in this population. Over the years, it has been interesting to listen to men and women, who fight against a system that is trying to save their lives, like adolescents kicking against the 'brick mother', which Henri Rey referred to, managing to robustly contain the most violent outbursts.

I recall two occasions of such emotional eruptions on the ward. One situation involved a young adult around 25 years old referred to with a pseudonym 'Yusuf'. 'Yusuf' had a diagnosis of autism and was on an acute ward in London due to his mother reportedly finding it difficult to manage him. I spent a lot of time with the ward residents, treading carefully in their fragile and temporary ward-home environment. I was aware that I could arrive and leave as I pleased but that residents and staff could not. I had chosen to work a great deal with children, young people and adults with a diagnosis of autism, which was significant autism in relation to verbal and non-verbal communication difficulties. Currently, there is a proliferation of people seeking autism diagnoses, especially amongst young people, where there does seem to be an element of social contagion about this need for a diagnosis, perhaps like a fashion accessory item. Parents can also want to diagnose their children rather than face the difficulties in themselves, paying psychiatrists enormous amounts of money to distract the problem to their children. Yet when informed about working with people with autism, it really is a matter of modifying one's own communication style and approach to accommodate the differences. Many are, however, adamant that the cause is genetic, and such a strong position needs to be assessed.

Returning to 'Yusuf', I was aware, in my countertransference, of rage within him, common amongst individuals with autism and learning difficulties due to the bullying they endure alongside being misunderstood. I learned from the nurses by way of handover that Yusuf's mother visited him to collect his benefit book, which she would then withdraw and not allow him access to. It was considered a safeguarding issue that this was occurring, likely being exploited financially and emotionally. As a young man who was perhaps little understood at school, he had fewer verbal communication skills than most and was likely being exploited by his mother, this would understandably lead to an inevitable accumulation of frustrations, hurts and anger. After his mother visited on the ward, his behaviour became alarmingly erratic and unsafe, charging around the ward, into people and objects.

On one memorable occasion, 'Yusuf' started trashing the living area, ripping the wires out of the ward TV from the wall and from the public-style telephone. He smashed the very fortified glass between the nursing station and the ward and smashed anything in sight. His pent-up rage was something to bestow, out of control, sudden and alarming. Security nurses were called, but by the time they arrived minutes later, 'Yusuf' had entered into the dining area, with reinforced glass windows between it and the rest of the ward. He managed to lock himself into this area and started thrashing against the walls and glass, managing to break through the thick glass; the lack of containment available to him in this state was frightening to observe. Just as 'Yusuf' was leaving through the glass window, the riot police arrived, an army of men, who crashed through the door with bulletproof shields and managed to capture him just in time as he stepped out of the smashed window. He could have lost his life in this state of mind, causing harm to himself and others. I ponder on how one person's anger can take 16 riot police and multiple hospital security staff to contain. Surely, this escalation could have been prevented. I was shocked, also because I spent a lot of time with 'Yusuf' playing games and doing arts and crafts and still remain saddened that such individuals are so easily exploited. On the other hand, it is understandable that not being fully oriented to verbal communication, being abused by his mother and misunderstood and likely talked about in his presence as if he wasn't there, would evoke great anger. An accumulation of frustrations, hurt and anger over many years clearly leads to such outbursts, and we need to think about how to do things differently. We need to act on observations of abuse in families of vulnerable people quickly; there is no excuse not to. Too few of us act on safeguarding matters straight in front of us, and too many organisations and individuals turn against people who report safeguarding matters. The UK has a very long way to travel until safeguarding is properly managed. Too many people turn a blind eye to harm being perpetrated. Why? It has been found that pedophiles are the most likely in court to be let off by a jury due to their charismatic personality style, propensity to lie in such a convincing manner and people's inability to face the reality that such horrific crimes as sexual abuse could be happening in their household or next door. Pedophiles seem to me to be steps ahead of most people and, therefore, are able to manipulate them. Having said this, pedophiles need help but are very resistant to it making a difference, likely due to their personality structure.

Another example of extreme patient behaviour occurred at a London hospital, where a female patient barricaded herself into the dining area and had two knitting needles. If this had been during the day, I can imagine that the ward manager would have managed to stand by her and talk to her, then ask her to hand over the knitting needles, as he had demonstrated doing numerous times before with hammers, axes, knives, scissors, nooses, alcohol and unprescribed drugs. On this evening occasion, the nurses didn't try to communicate with the patient but called the police. Fifteen offices arrived, cornering the woman and managing to regain control of the knitting needles.

It appeared over the top and, by all accounts, an unnecessary cause of distress to the patient and a waste of taxpayers' money and everyone's time. On so many occasions, I have wondered why nurses sound their alarms so readily rather than remaining calm and talking to the patient, which would likely work in such instances. Presumably, nurses and other staff could be trained in communication skills in order to prevent such unnecessary escalations, where one wonders whose childhood drama is being played out. Offering a still, calm presence on the wards is the best gift that can be offered to very frightened, chaotic and disorientated adults, whose child part is, at this point, usually in frenzied crisis and, therefore, in need of reassurance.

One of the saddest situations I have encountered was on a male acute ward, where a man there was very thought disordered due to his mental health issues and crack cocaine use. He had authorised permission for his universal credit to be handed over to his drug dealer to take charge of it. The man's dealer then had full control of his income, giving him crack cocaine, but was also supposed to leave him money for food, which did not happen. On numerous occasions, this man had regained mental capacity in the ward, promising staff that he would not allow this to happen again. However, he was unable to stand by this safeguarding agreement and refused to allow any details about the drug dealer to be shared. When the male patient was asked why he did this, he sadly responded that he didn't care if he lived or died.

When working on the acute wards, there is a safety protocol to follow, including gaining a handover from the nurse in charge, which was invariably brief and didn't generally include all the risks adequately, and this may be understandable considering the wards had 30 beds to cover in the handover. Nurses work hard and are on the frontline for long shifts daily on low pay. It was often difficult to understand what was being said for other reasons and was sensitive to address. I then secured an alarm to my belt after testing that it worked and signed into the ward, asking permission to enter. I was aware that the ward was the temporary home environment of over 30 individuals and their fragile place of safety for now. Most of the patients didn't want to be there, and frustrations and anxieties would frequently escalate into shouting and fights. Everyone needed to be safeguarded. Often, fights would break out, and I would see nurses or nursing assistants not intervening. And in this way, patients intervened, acting as staff, putting themselves at risk. At times, there were no nurses on the ward. They were either huddled in the nursing station or on a break. Menzies-Lyth observed and wrote about the coping mechanisms on wards to manage anxieties, such as this and the defences that are employed by frontline staff to manage their own feelings of exposure and fear. Nurses and other medical staff can appear harsh and aggressive, perhaps overwhelmed and losing touch with themselves, or, conversely, shut down as a defence. The cost of this, however, is losing contact with people as human beings and then being perceived as threats to be kept out.

I was aware that as a volunteer (I also worked on wards in a paid capacity), I could enter onto and leave the ward, whereas the nurses were there for long shifts within a different paid contract. The patients could not leave, and both of these elements set up the potential for resentments and hostilities towards me. Furthermore, patients were often not sure who I was and either perceived me as a doctor or social worker and were suspicious and guarded, at first, to talk to me. I learned to introduce myself to as many on the wards as possible, showing people my NHS badge and clearly stating that I am a volunteer who doesn't make any notes and is not part of the regular team. I spoke to all the patients on the ward to gather their views on topics to cover in the group and which kind of group, therefore, they wanted. From what the patients asked for, I organised a schedule for the group, and they named it, therefore, taking ownership of it, alongside specifying and agreeing the ground rules. Before each group, I let every single patient know about the group, knocking on each bedroom door and waiting for a response on two corridors, to warmly invite them to the group. Sometimes, after knocking and hearing no response, nurses recommended I open the door with the keys given to me by the staff (if enough were available since staff often went home with them) finding individuals hiding behind beds with their mattresses on the floor, or once in a cupboard. I would also walk into situations where immediate help was needed, such as when a person was trying to hang themselves, self-harming, disoriented, in deep distress or needing assistance to express their needs while hearing voices and/or in a state of acute psychosis. One woman was snoring with her eyes wide open, but she needed help with her personal hygiene. Such situations take a few moments to work out what is occurring, and the best action in the patient's best interests.

The nurses were both wary about my role and curious about how I was holding conversations with inpatients, both individually and in groups. I shared my plans with the nurses for the group work, which had been risk-assessed. The nurses were invited into all groups and attended regularly, which was helpful since they knew the patients well. I recall being assigned a room to see patients in on a one-to-one basis, which had a window where everyone on the ward could look into, which was far from private but did offer some protection for me. The room was not soundproof and directly next to the communal ward area, where the television was on full volume and there was much lively arguing, fighting, screaming and shouting amongst the 30 patients and staff gathered there. Additionally, nurses kept entering the room (called 'quiet room') to bring patient medication and ensure that they take it, which is understandable, but it struck me that there was really nowhere on the ward where patients had any privacy. This reminded me of Foucault's panopticon regarding his views on discipline and control, posed as a means to illustrate the proclivity of disciplinary contexts to subjugate the population. Foucault illustrates the prisoner of a panopticon as being on the receiving end of asymmetrical surveillance, where, in this context, the patient is seen, but he does not necessarily see and is an object of information but not a subject in communication. Those watching cease to be separate from those being watched (Foucault, 1977). Everyone was being watched on the ward, but there were different categories of power regarding whose word would be believed most. As can easily be imagined, the ward received numerous complaints from the patients, and remaining objective in a sea of accusations may have been difficult.

It would be reasonable to consider that the nurses on the wards who worked every day with patients may feel slighted by me holding one to ones with patients and with the skills I brought to the ward, which nurses had not been trained in. The ward manager was keen for me to work with the patients and help them, which was encouraging and supportive. I felt that the ward manager and psychiatrist and nurses invested a lot of trust in me, and their trust was respected throughout. I was very careful in all ways with the patients with whom I had contact. Nurses are starting to be trained in counselling skills which is a very positive move, in my opinion. Increasingly, I observed nurses holding consultations with the patients and having more verbal, supportive contact with them. However, I recall that a nurse had been assigned as a one-to-one support for a patient who was suicidal and at risk from other patients, and when I approached her bedroom door to invite her to the group, the nurse was sitting with the door closed and texting on her phone. Perhaps nurses feel the weight of low morale and low pay while working on the wards, which leads them to disengage, forgetting the risk the patient poses and the need for direct observation by the staff member. I was quick to check that the patient was okay. I was aware that the architectural shape of the wards, especially those based on old, institutionalised models, were usually two corridors of bedrooms with an L-shape which was more hidden, behind which the nurse was placed in this instance. I recall feeling angry that she wasn't offering the patient the care needed and that the patient literally could have taken her own life behind that closed door. This brought to mind the question of why nurses become carers and what they bring with them to the role. Increasingly onwards, there are nurses as patients. I also needed to not jump to conclusions since I did not know more than what I saw in this instance.

The majority of nurses I observed were dedicated and compassionate, but I also saw verbal and physical aggression shown to patients, which I reported. Well-built male nurses did often help with managing the myriad dramatic scenes on the wards, but at times, this power was misused, especially on female wards, where there is such a sensitivity regarding why most of the patients are there – due to domestic violence by men and a range of sexual and physi-cal assaults, sex trafficking and childhood sexual abuses. On one particular female ward, the male ward manager demonstrated exemplary skills in rela-tion to positioning himself with women, at the same time, very much being on their side and able to manage them appropriately, fairly and safely. This man-ager's approach was to get alongside the female inpatient and speak calmly and humanely in order to help them feel safe and unthreatened to then reason with them, for example, to take an axe from their hands. Time and again, I saw this approach working well for everyone's safety and well-being, with the least confrontation and the most respect and dignity shown. This not only further protected the staff-patient relationships but also supported ongoing healthier lives leading up to discharge, which is surely the most important factor.

## Restraint

It is necessary to consider the function of restraint for male and female inpatients on acute psychiatric wards. The Mental Health Act (2018) states that the restraint used must be proportionate both to the likelihood of the harm and the seriousness of the harm. It follows that the minimum level of restraint must be used; if the risk of harm diminishes, the restraint used must be reduced. It is further helpful to consider the function of restraint for hospital staff and the management structure. Physical restraint can be conceived of as an extreme response to managing someone's behaviour when they are in a mental health crisis. Reportedly, restraint can be experienced as humiliating, causing severe distress, and at worst, it can lead to injury and, sadly, even death. For example, in 1998, David 'Rocky' Bennett died at a medium-security mental health unit. Shockingly, since Rocky Bennett's death, there have been at least 13 restraint-related deaths of people detained under the Mental Health Act 1983. Eight of these occurred in a single year, namely 2011.

Physical restraint is primarily used for patients at risk of falling, those displaying motor unrest and agitated behaviour, and those who demonstrate an intention of causing harm to themselves or are at risk of suicide. The use of freedom-restraining measures and, particularly, the use of non-consensual physical restraints would be experienced as a serious intrusion of basic human rights and, as such, an act of violence against the patient. The improper use of physical restraints can cause injuries of varying severity, which can sometimes be fatal, as conveyed earlier. Mental Health Units (Use of Force) Act 2018 statutory guidance states the following:

## What is the use of force, why, and when can it be used?

The Mental Health Units (Use of Force) Act 2018 introduces the following definitions of use of force.

Use of force includes physical, mechanical or chemical restraint of a patient or the isolation of a patient (which includes seclusion and segregation).

The act defines the different types of force as follows:

- physical restraint: the use of physical contact which is intended to prevent, restrict or subdue movement of any part of the patient's body
- mechanical restraint: the use of a device which is intended to prevent, restrict or subdue movement of any part of the patient's body and is for the primary purpose of behavioural control
- chemical restraint: the use of medication which is intended to prevent, restrict or subdue movement of any part of the patient's body

The act states that isolation is any seclusion or segregation that is imposed on a patient. However, it does not define these terms. The definitions of these are provided in Annex A of the *Mental Health Act 1983*: code of practice, which applies to any patient in a mental health unit detained under that act, which defines them as follows:

- seclusion: the supervised confinement and isolation of a patient, away from other patients, in an area from which the patient is prevented from leaving, where it is of immediate necessity for the purpose of the containment of severe behavioural disturbance, which is likely to cause harm to others
- (long-term) segregation: a situation where, in order to reduce a sustained risk of harm posed by the patient to others, which is a constant feature of their presentation, a multi-disciplinary review and representative from the responsible commissioning authority determines that a patient should not be allowed to mix freely with other patients on the ward on a long-term basis

These definitions are broadly consistent with definitions which relate to the use of force set out in the Health and Social Care Act 2008 (Regulated Activities) Regulations 2014 ('the 2014 Regulations') and in the Mental Health Act 1983: code of practice.

'Chapter 26: Safe and therapeutic responses to disturbed behaviour' of the Mental Health Act 1983: code of practice provides further statutory guidance in relation to the use of force, which staff are under a statutory duty to have regard to in relation to patients in mental health units detained under the Mental Health Act 1983.

In particular, paragraphs 26.36 and 37 provide further guidance on the meaning of restrictive interventions (use of force):

deliberate acts on the part of other person(s) that restrict a patient's movement, liberty and/or freedom to act independently in order to:

- take immediate control of a dangerous situation where there is a real possibility of harm to the person or others if no action is undertaken, and;
- end or reduce significantly the danger to the patient or others.

Restrictive interventions should not be used to punish or for the sole intention of inflicting pain, suffering or humiliation.

Where a person restricts a patient's movement, or uses (or threatens to use) force then that should:

- be used for no longer than necessary to prevent harm to the person or to others;
- be a proportionate response to that harm, and;
- be the least restrictive option.

It is important to acknowledge that there are circumstances where it may be difficult to avoid the use of force to ensure the safe care and treatment of the patient, and the safety of other patients and staff. For example, nasogastric feeding for patients with eating disorders or a need to restrain a patient with dementia who is resisting or refusing help with personal care and support. Even within these situations it is still essential that the relevant legal principles are applied and that the use of force is proportionate.

In a significant study (Berzlanovich et al., 2012), there were 26 cases of death while the individual was physically restrained in hospital settings. Three of these cases involved patients who died of natural causes while restrained (requiring further investigation), and one was a suicide. The remaining 22 deaths were caused solely by physical restraint – all of which occurred in patients under nursing care who had not been continuously observed. The immediate cause of death was strangulation (11 cases), chest compression (8 cases) or when in the head-down position (3 cases). In 19 of these 22 patients, the restraints were incorrectly fastened, including two cases in which improvised nonstandard restraints were used. One nursing home patient died because of an abdominal restraint, even though it had been correctly applied. She was mobile enough to slip through the restraint until it compressed her neck and then was unable to extricate herself from it, resulting in death by strangulation.

In what is stated earlier, the emotional aspect of restraint, which consciously or unconsciously is sought out by the patient, is considered. Having witnessed many incidents of restraint, it seems that physical holding, usually by a large group of security nurses, also offers an observable sense of the patient being held in mind and emotionally contained. On the acute wards in North London, I noticed one patient repeatedly behaving badly to gain restraint and spoke about needing it to 'gain some attention rather than none' and 'I haven't been held much in my life'. Often, when undergoing therapy work with children, it becomes clear that negative attention, in whatever form this takes (physical, sexual, emotional and verbal violences), is better than being ignored. I think that individuals used to such negative attention become habitually used to being treated this way, through learning from experience and then seeking out similar negative attention elsewhere, including on wards in a secure setting.

Restraint may serve the additional purpose of helping the patient manage distress, such as a patient who, having been told that she was HIV positive, found herself understandably so distressed that six large male nurses held her down whilst administering a sedative via injection into her upper arm. Nurses often did not want me to observe restraints, which intuitively raised a concern for me. I think that an aspect of this was genuine protection of the patient and myself. I have also witnessed restraints that were necessary in the circumstances of patients being very acutely unwell and out of control, particularly when attempts on life were demonstrated or when there was harm to others or from others. Lives have been lost through restraint, which is unacceptable and extremely painful to witness, especially the sorrow and loss experienced by family members under these circumstances. Thinking about the organisational dynamics of fatality through restraint can only lead to a view on the perpetrator as sadistic, prejudiced and out of control – clearly unsafe to be working anywhere near vulnerable and acutely distressed individuals.

Bringing the previous study up to date, an NHS Trust has made recent efforts to reduce restraint on their acute wards, alongside deeming it mandatory for staff to undergo training. Olaseni Lewis, a 23-year-old British man, died on 3 September 2010 at a south regional hospital after police subjected him to prolonged physical restraint. Lewis had voluntarily sought care following the onset of acute mental health issues and died from cerebral hypoxia (lack of oxygen to the brain) soon after, following actions that involved 11 officers of London's Metropolitan Police. After seven years of campaigning by Lewis's family and two enquiries by the Independent Police Complaints Commission (IPCC), a second coroners' enquiry was raised.

The enquiry ruled that the restraint was disproportionate and found the officers had failed to follow the training on both the restraint of people with medical conditions and treatment of non-responsive people. The relevant hospital was also judged to have had several failures in Lewis's assessment, treatment and care. The IPCC recommended a review of six police officers for gross misconduct in relation to the incident, but all were later cleared by the Metropolitan Police in closed hearings, which is extremely concerning. The NHS Trust received no charges, though it made changes to its internal processes as a result. How this left Seni Lewis's family feeling is difficult to think about.

The Mental Health Units (Use of Force) Bill 2018, known as 'Seni's Law', was passed into British law in November 2018, making several provisions to limit the use of force on mental health patients and to require police officers working in mental health units to wear police body cameras where this was considered reasonable. It also required that hospitals record data and release reports on incidents involving physical force, including data on age, gender and ethnicity of those restrained. All reports covering patient deaths must be reviewed by the Secretary of State in an annual review. The law is not in force yet. Seni Lewis's death returned to national attention in 2020, following the George Floyd protests in the United Kingdom, in relation to the disproportionate number of black, Asian and minority ethnic people killed by UK law enforcement officers. As stated previously, male acute wards are often very fragile environments, with violence breaking out frequently. The risk of working on such wards draws the nurses together, who are necessarily dependent on each other as a protective team. It is disappointing when a dangerous staff member is in the mix and the risk this brings to everyone.

Some patients are at risk from other patients, and there are multitudes of examples of assault from patient to patient on a daily basis. The process of sibling transference has helped clarify some of the aggressive interactions observed. As referred to previously but to elaborate on, the male patient gave his drug dealer direct authority over his universal credit payments who was supposed to allow the patient money for food. However, this had not happened. When he shared this with me, I was curious why he did this and his response was that he didn't care if he lived or died. The patient had been helped with skills to manage his money differently, but once he had disconnected from the drug dealer and regained control of his benefit money, within a week, he had set up the same situation with one of the patients on the ward who was selling crack cocaine to the inpatients. Once uncovered, this situation was easily addressed by ward nurses. However, I wondered about the attachment style being communicated here, where he deliberately put in control a person who would feed him drugs and not be able to break away from this. The patient returned to the ward repeatedly over many years, as inevitably, his health deteriorated from such an extremely unhealthy lifestyle.

Working with the most vulnerable men and women on acute wards, those displaying some of the most odd yet fascinating, eccentric and, at the same time, concerning behaviours have been brought by the police usually or voluntarily, or by concerned family and/or friends, to the place of safety, as described earlier. The secure ward offers an often life-saving space for people in the most acute and suicidal states of mind to gradually become calmer and, when relevant, sober up. Medication is perhaps the cornerstone of psychiatry, and acute wards are placed in psychiatric and medical model settings. Therefore, the first course of treatment on acute wards is medication, usually anti-psychotic medication, following an assessment of the individual's situation, assisted hugely on ward rounds by nursing staff notes and observations since the nurses are around the patients 24/7. Many psychiatrists perhaps come to learn about the limits of psychiatry and train in psychoanalysis or medical psychotherapy.

It is now pertinent to turn to look at a number of case studies where working with often remarkable male and female inpatients helps us learn profoundly about humanity, which could easily be overlooked or dismissed as nonsense. On the contrary, I consider that there is a wealth of opportunity to learn about how the mind works, when observing and working therapeutically with individuals in severe states. The aim is always to ease their pain and restore a sense of self, functionality and an improved quality of life.

In the case studies that follow, informed consent has been received from the individuals involved to publish about them. Pseudonyms and other identifying features have been carefully thought about and allocated, so as to protect and respect each person's privacy and confidentiality.

# 5   Case study 1 – 'MJ' – a case of additional dissociation

'This above all, To thine own self be true, And it must follow, as the night the day, Thou canst not then be false to any man'.

*Hamlet* – William Shakespeare

'MJ' is 45 years old, single, Asian-born and UK-raised from the age of 2 years old, highly intelligent, a trained scientist at an elite British university, alongside being a proficient musician and rock climber. He is a handsome, medium-built, brown-skinned male. His dress reflects a unique, astute, trendsetting mentality, aligned with a sharp-thinking inventor. MJ has entered inventions into high-profile competitions and won prizes for his designs. He is creative, softly spoken, empathic and sensitive to others' feelings, quiet yet observant, kind yet full of possibly unrecognised rage, spending large amounts of time on his own and not socialising with others, although sociable when spoken to. The multitude of medications which 'MJ' consumes daily includes clozapine, lamotrigine, sodium valproate, amisulpride, atorvastatin and sertraline. MJ managed to share that this medication appears to have helped with some symptoms of agitation, withdrawal, mutism, alcohol consumption and food intake, but it appeared to me that his quality of life is limited, particularly socially, although reportedly much loved and liked by those who know him. However, MJ doesn't initiate contact with others apart from those who visit the family home. 'MJ's opinions and observations are astute, and he considered his non-epileptic seizures began when he started the course of clozapine. It is apparent that MJ has always been socially phobic, reaching back to early primary school, where he reported to his mother repeatedly that he had not spoken to anyone else that school day.

## Background

MJ is the youngest of 3, with an elder sister, 'Akari', by 18 months and elder brother, 'Kaito', of 4.5 years. Both of MJ's parents are the youngest siblings in their families and are of very similar ages, leading to a seemingly close identification by them both with MJ. MJ's mother is elder to her husband by

DOI: 10.4324/9781003509059-6

ten months. The family moved to the UK at MJ's age of 2 years old due to MJ's father's promotion in an Asian-based media. His elder sister, 'Akari', with whom he is emotionally close, is lively, well-educated, divorced, diagnosed as gifted and talented and ambitious. Akari works in media and is hardworking and astute. She appears to attract envy from others, which is a struggle for her, but she is alert to presentations of truth as deceit.

When MJ was 22.5 years old, he reported in therapy that his elder brother, Kaito, who had become dependent on 'uppers and downers' – initially through his mother – and had been psychiatrically hospitalised a few times, went missing and never returned. He later died mysteriously, following an argument with his father, Kenzo. In this argument, Kaito had expressed needing to talk to his father about wanting to 'move on'; his father, being busy with work, had asked Kaito to wait. Kaito was last seen leaving the family home in a highly agitated state of mind. Kaito's loss devastated the family. His mother, Eml, never recovered from the loss of her son, the hurt always just under the surface and barely able to be talked about, without evoking choked tears.

In previous years, MJ shared with me that he had been hospitalised in the same ward as his elder brother, Kaito, both suffering with paranoia, hearing voices and experiencing delusions. Kaito is described as highly intelligent and ahead of his time, an excellent artist and a sociable, handsome, lively and fun loving character, who was well-read and inquisitive about the world. Kaito was considered popular with a large group of friends and romantic partners of whom he was fond.

This sudden death was devastating for MJ and his family, the siblings close-knit and caring towards one another. When Kaito had gone missing, the parents and MJ went on holiday, leaving Akari at home, who wanted to be there for Kaito when she thought that he would return home. Sadly, Akari received the news of her elder brother's death and had to try to track down her parents' whereabouts, inform them about what had happened and wait for them to return. Her then boyfriend had taken time off work to stay with her; Akari had understandably been in deep shock. One may wonder if the holiday was a deliberate attempt to avoid responsibility of Kaito's disappearance and death, then focused on Akari, who, unbeknownst to her at the time, wanted to wait at home in the hope that her brother would return alive, which was sadly not the case.

**Family dynamics**

MJ managed to share with me in therapy that his mother, Eml, is an Asian, sensitive, creative, introverted and very intelligent professional person, the youngest child of six – an eldest brother and four elder sisters – in a home of social workers, where Eml felt she did not have enough space and spoke little as a result, until she managed to leave home to attend training college in another northern Asian city. Here, her confidence grew, and she met her husband. Eml's father had volunteered to go into the army during World War

II, but this had not been mandatory, and from her age of 0–6 years old, her father was, therefore, absent. When Eml's father returned, he quickly became a director, working long hours to provide for his family. Three family generations lived in a small semi-detached home, where the children, Eml being one of them, had to share beds to sleep due to lack of space. The family were academically bright, and several of the male members, including the eldest brother and cousins, attended a top university, mainly studying languages, then working for the intelligence service and later becoming professors and lawyers. The female siblings became social workers and mothers. Eml was brought up in a small, rural Asian town and was keenly astute about people and money. She was very attached to her father, who died by a heart attack at his age of 54 in the car park of the organisation he directed. This appears to have had a devastating impact on Eml's life, finding it difficult to allow people to be separate from her – anxious, lacking confidence and believing that she needs people to help her in her life. Eml had been very close to her father.

MJ shared in therapy that Eml's mother, Aimi, raised six children during the Second World War, at a time when there were no washing machines and daily tasks needed to be managed single-handedly, whilst her husband was away in the army. Therefore, Aimi was a strong woman but distanced herself from her children by spending time in the kitchen cooking, washing and ironing clothes and doing other household tasks. There was a coldness, which perhaps emerged as a single mother of six. She favoured her only son, and he was the one who went to the top university early, but due to his character, he married a woman who told him what to do and devastated the family due to her mental illness and cruelty. Aimi's brother had died by drowning in the family bath, leaving Aimi, two sons and his wife behind.

Eml's upbringing, according to MJ, appeared to have been amidst a jam-packed home in a small Asian town, with other family members living in the same street, where they were frequently in and out of each other's homes. The family home was described as like an arguer cooker, claustrophobically hot, tensions rising and falling, with little or no space to be, with a strong pecking order amongst the siblings with everyone trying to be heard. Eml, on the one hand, was bullied, being the youngest, and, therefore, was unhappy but was also included in the sibling 'teasing'. The eldest brother appeared to have stepped into the father's role to control his five sisters, at his mother's command.

MJ recounted to me in therapy that when Eml managed to leave the family home and her confidence rose, she started speaking more freely and, with her fun personality and good looks, attracted Kenzo whilst at training college, and they were soon to be married. Unlike Eml, who had never gone on holiday as a child with little spare money in the family, Kenzo was from a wealthy family, his father a financial entrepreneur and mother an actress from a leading Asian city. At their time of meeting, Kenzo's father had recently died of Alzheimer's disease, which was devastating in the context of losing his beloved yet seemingly harsh and emotionally cold father. The father had given all his inheritance to a care home manager, with nothing handed to Kenzo or his elder brother, Haruto. Kenzo's mother had died of lung cancer at his age of 14 years old. Kenzo frequently visited his mother in the hospital and then suffered from flashbacks akin to post-traumatic stress disorder, re-emerging when his son Kaito tragically died. Kenzo had spent his childhood mainly reading in bed, frequently ill with tonsilitis until he was successfully treated with penicillin. After this treatment, Kenzo was able to rejoin school life and sport.

MJ recounted in therapy how his father, Kenzo, had attended a preparatory junior school, where the headmaster was reportedly a pedophile and had assaulted Kenzo at his age of 7 years old, who was unable to tell anyone until much later, when he recounted this experience to his daughter, Akari, who was understandably very concerned for her father, who would not allow her to offer him comfort. Kenzo minimised the incident, leaving Akari on her own with this experience not knowing what to do with it. Kenzo's brother, Haruto, had attended at an elite British university to read history, then became a stage manager amidst alcohol reliance, an eating disorder and possible bipolar disorder. Haruto had mood swings and depressive states, at times found by his family sitting in silence in a darkened room. Haruto additionally struggled with a restrictive eating disorder, possibly linked to his theatre role and focus on appearance; his was immaculate. Haruto appeared reliant on the more practical Kenzo for a home, with whom he stayed for over 30 years, when his relationship with a famous and beautiful film actress ended devastatingly. Haruto appeared nastily envious of his brother Kenzo's family and life, appearing to seek to undermine this in a sibling rivalrous way, persuading Kenzo to move the family nearer to him, then three weeks later, turning up on their doorstep homeless and distraught. This put Kenzo in a near-impossible situation, where he could hardly say no to his brother, Haruto. The family had not even had the chance to reconvene as a family in their new home when Haruto entered in. It seems that Haruto brought very difficult feelings into the family home, which was fragile, unsettled and grieving the loss of their home country and all their associated attachments of family, friends and familiar places. Haruto's feelings seemed to split the family apart.

MJ shared with me in therapy that due to Kenzo's job, the family had moved home a lot, causing disruption to being able to make friends and feel settled in one place for the children, creating a risk of vulnerability to them. With Asian attributes, MJ, Kaito and Akari faced challenges of being accepted into the school group. Akari was reportedly the only one in the family who adjusted her accent to fit in with her peers. She led on the lessons in her state primary school, then being ahead of most, at her next private all-girls school, where she was put down by her affected class counterparts, gaining high scores in her exams. MJ attended a well-known preparatory school and private secondary school, excelling in science and being awarded prizes for this. He was accepted at all the top universities for which he applied to study science. When studying chemistry on a degree course which had been overstretched by twenty per cent, MJ reported suffering a breakdown and had to return to his parents' home, from where he had been studying and never returned to complete the course. He lived on £25 a week when studying, a recollected added strain for him, yet his parents were wealthy. This raised questions regarding who was controlling the money flow in the family. It seemed that the father laid claim to the finances, yet not providing for his families basic needs was striking.

In therapy, MJ spoke about that once Akari had left home at age 17, to study in the North of England, which she had enjoyed, Kenzo came to collect her, nearly insisting that she come home. It seemed that Kenzo exerted a lot of control over family members, manifesting in their vulnerability, by him insisting on taking and collecting them by car, answering questions asked of others without their consent, setting the rules about what can and can't be talked about (nothing personal but politics and sport were acceptable) and smashing glasses out of the blue, keeping everyone on edge, coping with his shifting moods. It seemed that he suffered with PTSD. By disempowering his family members in these ways, they became more dependent and unable to leave him or do tasks for themselves. In Kenzo's early life and teenage years, he had experienced a lot of loss and abandonment, anxiety perhaps underpinning a need to control family members in this way, to ensure they don't leave and to manage his anxieties.

Kenzo, as reported by MJ in therapy, had insisted that he was a liberal parent, being naked in the family home when MJ, Kaito and Akari were young children. Akari asked her mother to stop her father from being naked in front of her at her age of 4–5 years old, since she didn't like it, but he continued. Akari spoke to her mother again about this, and he then stopped. Although Kenzo claimed he had a happy childhood, it was clear that there was a great deal of pain: his father appeared to treat his sons very harshly, whereas he spoilt females, in contrast. Kenzo's father behaved similarly, causing great hurt to his sons, who were sensitively intelligent. Kenzo bullied Eml, who was vulnerable. MJ was also shaken and rageful by their constant bullying of one another, which he was exposed to.

Kenzo had suffered from seemingly physical illnesses throughout his childhood, and one wonders to what extent this was linked with the pedophile headmaster at his preparatory school, which would naturally be extremely distressing. Shortly after Kenzo's mother died, his father met a care home manager in a bar, then leaving Kenzo and Haruto largely to their own devices. Kenzo joined the paratroopers, offering him security, a surrogate family and learning. He then gained employment in media, being quickly and frequently promoted, meaning the family moved often, adding vulnerability in an unsettled state. Kenzo appeared to be highly intelligent, and it seems that his elder brother, Haruto, was very competitive with him. Haruto was a scholar from an elite university, yet more academic and less able to manage day-to-day practicalities.

## MJ's life

The following personal information was shared in twice-weekly therapy with me over a ten-year period to date. MJ's sharing with me in therapy is held with deep respect regarding it being an immense privilege to share in someone's life in this way. A referral was made from the inpatient team to me for individual and family therapy work with the aim of facilitating improved communication about MJ's needs. I had worked on the ward where MJ had been sectioned, and a great deal of thought was given to managing the transition of boundaries from hospital to private therapy. Having been born at the family home in Asia, MJ was the youngest of three children. He was moved to the UK at his age of 2 years old, where the family stayed with Eml's mother, whilst securing their home in a small village. Here, MJ was reportedly a colic baby, requiring a lot of attention, especially at night. Kenzo had historically spent a lot of time working away from the family, seemingly too sensitive to manage family life, often reading a newspaper when in the home and finding it hard to become more involved. The newspaper clearly kept others out like a skin. He preferred Eml to not work, but she was bright and needed further occupation, then having to hide from Kenzo that she was working as a supply social worker. Eml had become pregnant many times but had sought termination, since she would be left to look after the children with little support from Kenzo, apart from financially.

MJ appeared a loner at school, telling his inquisitive mother that he had not spoken with any other child during his schooldays. MJ appeared very bright and made more friends at his prolific public secondary school but was introverted, a thinker, an engineer, an inventor. From the age of 13 years old, MJ reported creating gadgets all around his bedroom, one for turning on the main light without leaving his bed, another to turn the music on, another to dim the lights and so on and so forth. MJ then took over the loft space where Haruto had stayed amidst asbestos when recovering emotionally and psychologically from his marriage break-up, creating a disco there with his male friend, with whom he developed a homosexual relationship for several years, unbeknownst to his family. None of his family were aware of this relationship, although he told his sister, Akari, years later.

There appears to have been a close relationship between MJ and his mother, both scientifically and creatively minded, both the youngest in their family and both highly sensitive people. Once living in the UK, having moved several times due to Kenzo's work, the family home was gradually refurbished from a dilapidated state, and lodgers rented rooms amongst the family. Kenzo was away, working a lot. Haruto, whose moods were up and down, stayed in the home whilst working. Haruto knew all the famous theatre and film actors and directors, alongside his ex-wife's contacts. Haruto was an avid reader of plays. His good looks and immaculate presentation attracted attention. He ate alone in his brother's home, drank alcohol secretly and demonstrated excess in his exercise, linked to weight control and self-esteem.

MJ's elder brother, with whom he had an, at times, strained relationship, attended a state secondary school, where he appeared to become involved with non-prescribed drugs. There was tension between the two brothers, partly because Eml appeared to identify with MJ, paying him extra attention, for example, in helping him with his homework since MJ is partially blind and has a diagnosis of dyslexia. Many hospital appointments had been arranged with surgery to try to find a solution for his reduced sight. Eml's eyesight was similarly hindered and her learning style slower but thorough. During MJ's early teens, his elder brother, Kaito, who had a large group of lively friends from the same street, started to withdraw. The family home was as Kenzo prescribed, 'Free for all. Help yourself', and in the guise of liberal parenting, MJ and his siblings were left unruly and vulnerable. Kenzo would undo the rules that Eml put in place, undermining her authority.

MJ shared with me in his therapy how the family home became locally known as a place where everyone could go to drink alcohol, smoke cannabis and other recreational drugs, with no boundaries I place due it seemed to denial. Eml appeared blind to it. Although she tried to instil rules, Kenzo, her husband, undid them and allied with Akari against Eml, which Akari deeply regretted, when she later understood the bullying pair she had become drawn into. Kenzo spent large amounts of time away working. Kaito appeared to be involved in taking various drugs and became very agitated, depressed and paranoid. Kenzo did not recognise the importance of developing one's own identity during adolescence and shouted at Kaito to change his experimental clothes in front of his friends and, in this way, frightened and humiliated him, which extended to some of his friendship group bullying and mocking Kaito. There appeared to be no secure home for Kaito, whose life had been uprooted at his age of 13 years old, from the countryside with established friends, to a UK capital and rough secondary state school. Having taken unprescribed medication through his mother and insensitive input from his father, Kaito became psychiatrically unwell. With Kenzo and Eml busy with their work and life, would sneak medication into his food and drink, which devastated trust. On the other hand, they may have been at a loss as to what to do.

Reflecting on the family dynamics as a therapist, Kenzo, through no fault of his own, seems to have been a vulnerable child who perhaps experienced an identity crisis. He was terrified by a pedophile headmaster, had no support for this, became ill with persistent tonsilitis and missed out on school and all its social aspects. As a handsome man, he had a great deal of wanted and unwanted attention from men and women alike. In the army, he experienced his fair share of unwanted homosexual attention and perhaps reacted vehemently, possibly triggered by the early pedophile headmaster's approaches towards him in his office. Kenzo had experienced further difficulties, such as the death of his parents when he was 21 years old and a seemingly anorexic and alcoholic brother, who went early to an elite British university to read a popular and, therefore, competitive subject and who was upheld as a 'scholar', likely leaving Kenzo in the shadows. Kenzo's father's treatment of his sons appears to be cruelly and emotionally harsh and painfully abandoning.

I reflected that the seeming narcissistic consequences for Kenzo's personality structure, which starts to dominate this narrative of MJ's therapy, was reportedly played out by Kenzo's solitary media existence, then mainly spent driving from one end of the UK to another. Kenzo's sensitivity, perhaps, made it difficult for him to be in the family. Eml had received a grammar school education, was a slow reader and was not a high achiever, though it seems this was due to a marked lack of confidence. Eml seemed to have a great deal of unprocessed hurt bubbling under the surface and was easily dominated by Kenzo, who could persuade and convince, but the content was often unfounded. Kenzo appeared so fragile that he undermined Eml and his offspring, almost like they were competitors in the workplace and, in this way, caused harm with what seems like underpinning unprocessed aggression and violence. Akari had brought a kitten home, which Eml and Kenzo had agreed to take in, but later, Kenzo kicked this cat, who shook in terror like the rest of the family, then the cat died. It seemed that there was a lack of consistent and reliable safe parenting from Kenzo, who could be seen as putting his children and family at risk, rather than protecting them, perhaps through PTSD.

I considered that it can be understood that Eml pushed Kenzo away due to his narcissistic tendencies, as Rey had envisaged to return to the 'marsupial pouch' of perceived safety of the mother, which may feel like one moving inside another's body for protection and maternal warmth. Kenzo found it almost impossible to allow others to have their own existence; he was highly intrusive into people's minds, perhaps feeling more acutely threatened by differences that challenged his own sense of self, as shown, for example, in his adamant responses to differing opinions. Kenzo's level of conviction in imparting information to persuade others to make a certain decision based on his needs was marked, seemingly further underpinned by the need to be right. This indicated a fragile ego and lack of confidence and perhaps cavalier approach to truth, which changed depending on who he was talking to. Matters about truth and reality raise difficult questions regarding who, if anyone, is in a position to make decisions about them, which is well-debated. Eml was instructed by Kenzo to put the three children to bed before he came home so that he had Eml's undivided attention. It seems that Kenzo's needs were prioritised much above those of Eml or their children. Kenzo was extremely possessive of Eml, who, to a certain extent, allowed it.

It seemed that Kenzo's sons and daughter were brutally and persistently emotionally attacked. It seems this was done to prevent them from posing a threat of competition to him, alongside maintaining them in a traumatised state. MJ, being bright, presumably posed an enormous threat to Kenzo, alongside his strong good looks and positive attention from Eml. Therefore, MJ and Kaito were far from encouraged to be independent since Kenzo created their learned helplessness by doing everything for them without teaching them the skills for independence. This created a disturbing situation where Kenzo became the best at everything (like his brother, Haruto, had), while others were disabled in turn to maintain Kenzo's position as the most competent. This behaviour may have been learned from his father and public school, where it was established that there was severe bullying of Kenzo. The emotional and financial neglect of Eml and their three children was difficult to comprehend. MJ bonded more with his mother out of survival, which appeared as co-dependence between them. This was further apparent as MJ became a stand-in husband when Kenzo, it seemed, slept due to his inability to face the world or reality. There was little emotional or physical support offered to Eml, who was essentially abandoned with three young children in various unfamiliar locations, whilst Kenzo was promoted, with work, becoming the focus of his life above all else. In this way, Kenzo gained financially, but this was not made available to the family, who wore tattered clothes and barely had enough to eat.

MJ shared with me in therapy that when he was 17 years old, he was working hard for his A levels, but his additional needs were not accommodated by the school. At this time, Kaito was part of a trendy, intelligent group of friends in the street where the family lived. Akari (MJ's sister) had developed bulimia nervosa, mainly caused by the emotional turmoil in the family and a school peer who encouraged her to lose weight. One night, at around 3 AM, Akari, who seemed to notice more of what was happening in the family, heard a loud smash. Thinking that there was a burglar downstairs, she found a cricket bat and cautiously but determinedly went down the stairs of the family home. She reported recalling hearing a surprised voice from the kitchen, 'It's not that big', as she followed a trail of blood droplets into the kitchen. Surprisingly, she saw her younger brother standing there, holding and looking at his cut left arm. Again, he said 'It's not that big a cut, is it?' Akari was shocked to see her younger brother so calm, speaking in this rational manner, whilst in front of her was a deep cut. Reportedly, she asked MJ, 'What happened, MJ?' He stood calmly, continuing to look at his deeply cut arm, blood slowly dripping from it onto the wooden floor. 'I put my fist through my bedroom window. I was trying to escape'. Akari concernedly enquired, 'You thought that you would escape through the bedroom window. Why not through the door? And escape from what?' Akari recalls feeling a mix of concern, anger, upset, disbelief and shock at what MJ was saying. Akari asked MJ to sit down and hold his arm straight upwards. 'I'm going to get Mum and Dad'.

MJ communicated to me further in therapy how Akari ran up the stairs, knocked on her parents' bedroom door and, hearing no response, knocked again. But again, with no response, she entered and gently roused her mother to respond, saying, 'You need to wake up. MJ has hurt his arm, and he needs to go to hospital'. From what seemed like a mock sleep, Eml said, 'What are you waking me up for? I need to go to work in the morning. You deal with it'. However, Akari's intuition led to persist in saying, 'You are his parents, and he needs you right now to help him. He has a deep gash on his arm by punching the window. He needs his parents'. Eml was angry and scoffed at Akari, who stood her ground. Akari was wondering, 'How can I get to the hospital at three in the morning?' 'You need to help him. He's down in the kitchen on his own. He needs your help. He needs his parents'. Eml responded, 'Okay,

I'll wake your father to deal with it. You go back down with MJ'. Akari was shocked and furious at the realisation of her mother arguing with her about taking responsibility and helping MJ, who was clearly in need. This made her wonder about her own safety, which felt perplexing. Her mother couldn't love her children. Akari returned to the kitchen, seeing her brother calmly tending to his wound. Akari waited and waited. She went back to her parents' bedroom, where her mother had turned over to go back to sleep. More determined, Akari stood over her mother, speaking more sternly to her to attend to MJ. She went and stood by her father and spoke loudly about the matter. He woke and then Eml said, irritated, 'For God's sake, I have to go to work early in the morning. I thought that you would help us on this occasion'. Akari said that she needed to go back to sleep, whilst Eml asked, 'What do you think we need to do? You've woken us up'. Akari sat with MJ, and around 15 minutes later, her parents appeared, when she could finally hand over the responsibility of her poor brother to them.

MJ shared with me, in therapy, that they drove off in the car, and the next day, she learned that MJ had been kept in the hospital since he stated that voices had instructed him to put his first through his bedroom window to escape. Thankfully, MJ had not gone through the window, which was a real potential risk. Perhaps MJ crashing his fist through the window and consequently no parents responding may highlight part of the underpinning difficulty. It was as if no parents were in the home, offering MJ and Akari this stark experience of absence and abandonment, at a time of such great need of protection, comfort and attention.

I met with MJ's family and then his parents on seven occasions in the ten years of therapy to date. Twice-weekly therapy continued between MJ and myself after he had been discharged from the acute ward. MJ managed to share that he had remembered a dream from the acute ward, and my notes from this session state the following:

A dove was resting on my mind, slightly covering my right eye and this annoyed me a bit. The white dove was trying to fly away but it was trapped and this was both beautiful and hopeful but also painful, annoying and frustrating. I could hear the dove's wings flapping loudly as it tried to fly away but moments later I realized it was still stuck, I suppose, to my mind (laughs).

At this time, I had been sectioned which lasted for two long weeks and I recall being very keen to leave and to go home but at the same time realizing that I was back wanting to escape from my family home, perhaps illustrated by the acute ward dream of the dove, I pondered. I realize that I have several challenges in my life, one being very weak eye sight, with an astigmatism which means that I have a wonky eye, which creates blurred vision and focusing on anything is very difficult. During schooling, no one had picked up on this but my mum kept trying

to get the message through to them and took me to umpteen eye special-
ists. I did struggle more than the other kids but did achieve some things.
I know that I was prone to bumping into objects such as lampposts,
which was embarrassing but also physically and emotionally painful
for me. I find it difficult to know where the steps are and this is really
difficult and I find myself falling over quite a bit. I also have a diagnosis
of dyslexia, alongside treatment resistant paranoid schizophrenia. I do
experience paranoia quite often which I don't think anyone understands
but it takes me out of reality and is very unpleasant. I don't want to talk
about my paranoia, it's all part of the paranoia, it not being easy at all
to talk about.

MJ shared with me in therapy how, during his teenage, his elder brother,
Kaito, had a large group of creative, trendy and good-looking friends but had
become involved in smoking pot and perhaps other non-prescribed drugs.
Kaito started becoming mentally unwell when MJ was around the age of
16 years old, perhaps a year prior to the incident with MJ having punched
the window. Through paying close attention in the therapy to what MJ was
conveying in his soft, gentle and insightful manner of speaking, it seemed that
there was a main difficulty in him and his siblings being helped to individu-
ate. MJ's brother, Kaito, had separated by becoming a volunteer fruit picker,
but no support was given to him, it seemed, by his parents to build a home.
Kaito reportedly had gone missing but was 'tracked down' living in a shed,
which the farmer and his wife had given to him, who had assumed that he
was destitute. Kaito had become mute and was living in isolation and a state
of neglect when his parents eventually managed to find him. In my countertransference, I deeply felt the sadness, anger and perplexity regarding how
parents could lose their children in this way, only to then spend time tracking
them down again. I considered that my countertransference resonated with
the patient's past abandonments and loss being repeated through their children, which is heartbreaking. From talking with Kaito's father, he shared that
he had similarly tried to find his brother when Haruto was at university and
found him lying alone, drunk in a meadow.

According to MJ's sharing in therapy, MJ's sister, Akari, was a lively and
bright character, again with a large group of friends who spent a lot of her
time with boyfriends and girlfriends, enjoying nights out and partying. MJ
was more of a quiet, introverted character and the parents' youngest, like
his parents, who perhaps were attached differently to him, compared to
Kaito and Akari. Akari had left the family at the age of 17 to attend a university course deliberately 300 miles away and had been greatly relieved to
gain respite from a family home, which appeared unpredictable due to her
mother's naivety, frustrations and denial, as well as her father's rigidity. Kenzo
had not received adequate parenting himself. He was a media entrepreneur
with extremely high intelligence but was brought up reportedly spoilt, and

therefore, the world needed to revolve only around his unmet needs, which is deeply saddening. He controlled his family and others to meet his (unmet) needs. Kenzo appeared to find difference to his mindset intolerable.

MJ recounted in therapy that he had had many encounters with the police since he heard voices instructing him to do various acts, such as escaping the country by stealing a car. He started the car using a metal coat hanger, which worked. However, MJ was spotted by police and pulled over, soon realising that he was in great distress and accompanying him home. Over the course of the therapy, lasting 15 years to date, it was worth considering the function of the police in this family's life over several decades, perhaps performing the paternal function of safety and/or the law of the father, as described by Lacan. Unconsciously, the two brothers, MJ and Kaito, found themselves on many occasions in contact with the police, and I wondered about the limit that this authority set for them. Kaito had been called to attend a magistrate's court once for trying to pay a child's fare on the bus. MJ managed to share with me that Kaito kept a log on the kitchen wall of amounts that he felt he owed his parents, especially his father, and would engrave on the wall small lines signifying the amount of money owed. The way money was used as a means of communication in this family, perhaps, highlighted how Eml and the three children were starved of comforts, whilst the father lived luxuriously in conference hotels and controlled the family finances.

There are many vivid descriptions of MJ's experiences, which spoke of family tragedy. MJ recounted in one therapy session the following (from my notes):

> My sister Akari and I were really quite close, often joking around because we were close in age by eighteen months. She used to always give me a piggy back when I was younger and tell me bedtime stories about Barney bear, my first teddy bear. My mother used to invite me on her dates, which must have been very annoying for Akari. I can see that (laughs), who would want their younger brother there but my mum made sure that I went. My sister moved after my dad collected her from the Midlands University. I don't think he wanted her out of his sight, it just seems very controlling now I look at it again with you. This space supports me to remember stuff from a long time ago. I remember Akari lived in a rundown flat, it was really very substandard, the landlord did not care clearly and I wonder how my parents were happy for her to live in such a horrible place, quite frankly. I visited her there like all the places she moved to. I think Akari suffered a lot because my dad didn't seem to be able to acknowledge anyone else's existence, including my mothers and there was no way that he could empathize or consider anyone else's needs, unless they impinged on his. Akari had to work all hours, whilst my dad had a huge bank account, I recall her walking around in rags and he never helped her out. My brother Kaito ended up

living in a bare shed on a farm, the farmer and his wife giving him more than my parents could, it is shocking to me thinking back. I noticed that if anyone gave me anything including respect, I was so starved for this that I went over the top and thanked them so much, their words filling such a gap inside me, is very sad. How I survived I really don't know and I am always thinking about my survival because I still haven't been able to escape.

Looking back again, when my sister was living in this squat type place just along from a famous nightclub, I remember going to the nearby station and looking in a lingerie shop in the station and thinking 'I should become a woman' and that if I were to buy the clothes that I saw and wear them, that I would need two iceberg lettuces to make up for the breasts that I didn't have. It was as if my mind had been taken over and was telling me to do these things. I didn't buy any of the lingerie but I must have intended to, since I turned up at my sister's flat carrying two iceberg lettuces, which she put in the fridge, not knowing why I had bought these but questioning what they were for and always acting respectfully towards me, she is a very loving sister. I used to call her 'my sist' but that was a long time ago (smiles) it's elder sister syndrome. I told Akari why I had bought the icebergs years later and she was interested and said it sounded like a beautiful idea but that I may be disoriented regarding my sexual orientation and identity. It was confusing for me.

Looking back, I feel compassion for myself, since I had been having a gay relationship with one of my friends, which none of the family knew about but it went on for seven years and a lot of the sex was in the family home. I suppose I realized that no one noticed. My sexuality was a source of immense disorientation for me, since my mother didn't seem keen on homosexuality, assuming that I was heterosexual and it was impossible to talk about anything personal with my parents. My father, I thought was homosexual, but hid this through being heterosexual but I may not be right about this but he had very strong responses to homosexuality which made me think he was. I see that he is a very good looking man, like my brother and mother. Akari always had a lot of male fans. My father talks about one boyfriend going out the back door, whilst one comes in the front door (laughs), Akari is a laff.

The image of the iceberg lettuce breasts is imaginative and phantastical, and at the same time, I explored gender identity and transgender phenomena with him. I wondered also about his own experiences of breastfeeding, and he was able to talk to his mother about this. I wondered if this experience was in some way a transgenerational communication. I enquired, and he recounted that his mother had kindly shared that she had developed arthritis or at least her hands had frozen when she was trying to breastfeed MJ and had had to ask her husband to return home from one of his many conferences to help her feed MJ. The impression is of MJ's mother having little emotional support from Kenzo. Apparently, Kenzo and Eml had discussed division of roles, whereby Eml looked after the children and Kenzo was the financial provider, but the different roles had perhaps become too compartmentalised. It seemed that perhaps the lack of emotional support from Kenzo, alongside his absences for whatever reasons, led to a subfamily emerging with different dependency needs being enacted. It sounds like Eml needed to keep Kenzo's possessiveness of her at bay, leading to him being ejected from the family home, ensuring more time for her children, which otherwise Kenzo would try to usurp. The skewed competitive relationships as perceived by Kenzo led him to act out reported emotional and psychological damage to his children and wife, including neglect. It seems that the extent of his self-interest was severe.

In another therapy session (MJ laying on the couch), he retold his need for escape, and I wondered what was being repeated rather than remembered and worked through, my thinking informed by Freud's astute observations expressed in his paper of the same name (Freud, 1914). MJ had described his confusion and vulnerability in many ways, and I certainly was aware of feeling maternal towards him in his plight. Waking up many times in the early morning and leaving the family home at 3 AM to steal a car to leave the country felt heartbreaking, at least because no one noticed his absence in the home and was suffering such difficult thoughts, 'hearing voices' (in quotation marks to try to understand what was meant by this in MJ's personal internal context). MJ shared the following with me, which was recorded in my notes:

> I thought that I was meant to leave the country and the way that I was going to do this was by boat. I went down to the riverside and walked along a while and found a boat and lay under the floorboards waiting to be taken out of the country. I lay there for what seemed like a long time but then heard the owner leave the boat and I thought that it must be the wrong boat and managed to leave. I went home thankfully but thought this was what I should do.

MJ told me in therapy that he had shared this with his sister, Akari, but no one else in the family. She had been very perplexed and concerned about her brother when she heard of this experience, as had I. MJ's elder brother, Kaito, also shared a lot with Akari, and I wondered about how the maternal function had been displaced to Akari, both of her brothers turning to share with her as to a trusted maternal figure. Perhaps, this dynamic emerged through Kenzo's possessiveness of Eml. MJ further informed me that Kenzo had managed to sever the relationship between Akari and Eml through persistent denigration of Eml and affirmation of Akari, who was a quick thinker and a reader, which pleased Kenzo. MJ recounted how painful this situation was to observe, leading to Akari developing bulimia nervosa and having to have veneers glued onto her teeth due to the erosion by the reflux stomach acid, following deliberate vomiting and laxative use.

I thought with MJ in therapy about his understanding of these repeated experiences of feeling that he was being told to leave the country, and together, we discussed the possibly of the unmet childhood needs of the parents being played out in a sadomasochistic way, pushing MJ out of the home in this compulsive and dangerous manner. Around the time of the boat experience, MJ had then felt he was to go to Portsmouth and that he would be taken out of the country that way. Thankfully, the police picked him up in Portsmouth and contacted his parents, who then went to collect him. My sense was that there were a lot of instances, especially involving Kenzo, where he took family members to places where they had little choice to say no, collecting them almost as if he were collecting parcels rather than treating them as his supposedly beloved family members. I couldn't help but wonder whether MJ's parents noticed that he had gone and, if they did, where they thought he was. MJ appeared to be starved of positive attention. MJ recounted an additional similar repeating escape phantasy that he acted out, as recorded in my notes:

I thought that if I went down the road to a particular antique shop on the high street, near to where we lived, that I could jump into one of the antique wooden chests that I had seen there and that the shop owner would cover me with oranges and cart me out of the country that way.

As a female therapist, I considered the sibling transference to me regarding his sister and recognised how much such positive reverberations can assist the therapeutic alliance, alongside the dual emotional poles of idealism and derogation. As a sister myself, with a close relationship to two brothers, interestingly mirroring MJ's sibling grouping, I reflected on this in supervision with Professor Robert Hinshelwood over the past 15 years. Professor Robert Hinshelwood had been a main encouraging factor in relation to my work with adults with schizophrenia, for which I am very grateful. It was possible to work through the less positive aspects of MJ's relationship with his sister, Akari, particularly his reference to her as a 'sist' (cyst) regarding her elder sister status and his dependence on her without the presence of another reliable and consistent parent to help him. To date, MJ's unmet needs limit his sister's life considerably. His family situation highlights such misinformed parenting, presumably due to similarly historical absent parenting in one form or another and for a possible plethora of reasons. I certainly feel compassion for MJ's parents and deep concern for MJ.

MJ informed me that he had, in fact, jumped into the wooden chest in an antique shop and that the owner had asked MJ to get out since I had wondered to what extent this recounting of experience was phantasy. MJ had been confused by the owner's response, which is understandable in such a convinced state of mind. Managing the sense of vulnerability in such a therapeutic dialogue was possible but interestingly led to a sense of aggression in my countertransference, which seems to be an accompanying emotion. This insight is informative of perhaps what is cut off for MJ, whose parents don't want to know about his anger, his mother perhaps too vulnerable herself to manage and his father perhaps not interested. My impression is that MJ's father had experienced a great deal of vulnerability all of his life and particularly during early adolescence, when he was exposed to his mother dying of cancer over a three-year period, therefore, since Kenzo was ten years old. Following this tragedy of Kenzo's mother dying young, MJ's paternal grandfather then abandoned his father and brother and met another woman who was described as a 'gold digger', taking advantage of his early dementia by all accounts and robbing MJ's father and brother of their inheritance; of main concern to Kenzo was the loss of personal photographs. The extent of Kenzo's vulnerability and hurt is difficult to think about, and he seems to have had to become so defended to the extent that he no longer could feel and, therefore, unaware of the hurt he then perpetuated. MJ was left yearning for a father figure, and his homosexuality seemed to perhaps serve the function of looking for this and finding mainly abusive older men, through various encounters in gay bars, which MJ had frequented. I was powerfully aware of how MJ was seeking the love that his father had not been able to provide for him, leaving MJ seemingly starving for attention. MJ's non-epileptic seizures gained much attention and time from his father; MJ finally gaining the attention he needed, but only possible in this way. The attention MJ's father then gave to him was sitting with MJ, mopping his brow, fetching toast and tea and talking with him.

MJ shared in therapy with me that he had left the family home in his late teens and early twenties to travel to a known central location to sit and drink tea from 2 to 5 AM in Burger King. I wondered if MJ was looking for male sexual partners or needed the space to think. Again, there was no mention of his family being aware of this, although he had shared about this with Akari.

MJ conveyed to me in therapy that he had gained positive A-level grades in science and was clearly gifted and talented in the subject. He was accepted unconditionally into top universities but unconsciously gave up the role of achiever when he had a breakdown, which again took him back home. Perhaps MJ's return home speaks of the difficulties between his parents. It seems likely that there was so much pressure placed on MJ away from home that it was inevitable for him to return due to the tensions in his parents' lonely marriage, requiring him as a stabiliser amongst other roles, such as surrogate husband. It appeared to be an unhappy marriage between MJ's parents, involving constant bickering and arguments, as well as threats from MJ's father to leave Eml, causing her great distress. Eml had gone through breast cancer and a mastectomy when Akari estranged herself from the family, following Kaito's tragic and sudden death. Akari saw no positive way forward in the family, mainly due to Kenzo becoming increasingly aggressive towards her, as she asserted more independence. Kenzo's 'accidental' violent acts, such as closing his boot on her hand, causing her great pain with blood drawn, indicated the need to flee. Also, at this time, strangely, Kenzo became the legal guardian to one of his goddaughters, and Akari felt pushed out understandably, as her half-cousin, Aki, was brought into the family with no discussion with MJ or Akari and seemingly replacing Kaito. Aki was extremely disturbed as an adopted daughter of Eml's brother, Akio, who was extremely bright linguistically but weak emotionally and who had, perhaps as a result of this weakness, married a psychopathic wife. Since Akio was away a lot working in 'intelligence', his two adopted children, including Aki and an additional blood child, were mistreated by his wife, a very needy, controlling person.

Reportedly in therapy, MJ had clearly experienced a series of traumas and seemingly gained no psychological support with them, partly, it seems, due to Kenzo being anti-therapy and communicating this not in a way that disallowed open discussion and choice but more as in a threatening, presumptive monologue. MJ had attended two sessions at a private clinic but didn't open up and felt that the clinician sat in silence, as did MJ. Kenzo started increasingly controlling more aspects of the family life, creating files on his children, claiming that his childhood had been all positive and blaming Eml for the ills in the family, such that he referred to her as 'murderess', in relation to Kaito's death, which she did not allow. MJ had lost his elder brother under tragic circumstances and then his sister left the family, and he did not know where she was, although she kept in touch with him when she could, as she was separating, saving her life and doing what she could to gain a home, something that her parents could not or would not provide for her.

From what MJ shared with me in therapy, it became apparent the extent of the threat imagined by MJ's parents – his mother in a lonely marriage, where her husband spent all of his time elsewhere. Kaito had divulged that he wanted to 'move on', but the meaning of this had not been adequately acted on by inept staff. Following this, Kaito's body had been found dead at the bottom of the river. The coroner's report was one of death by immersion (drowning). Eml heroically managed to face that she considered that Kaito had taken his own life, telling MJ that she had attended a meeting where it had been discussed that Kaito had stated that he wanted to take his own life. In this way, Eml was able to face reality but suffered from intrusive guilty thoughts of regret, perhaps obsessively so, leading to a sleepless life. Kenzo chose his own narrative around Kaito's death, claiming that he had experienced an epileptic seizure and fallen into the river. Kenzo blamed Eml for not having acted on the meeting content, which Kenzo had not attended.

It was very saddening for me to reflect on the tragic loss of Kaito, and its meaning in the family is obviously profound. Kaito had begun to recover from his anguish, but perhaps the contrast of how he felt and the spring months of March posed too much of a conflict for him. Or perhaps by recovering, he realised the loss of time and life for him posed an unbridgeable gap.

Spring is a risky season for those with suicidality.

MJ recounted in therapy with me how he managed to gain accommodation through his mental health and lived three miles away from his parents. Unfortunately, the threat of MJ's separation seemingly caused so much distress between his parents that they would not allow MJ any space to grow and develop as an independent entity. They phoned him repeatedly, disallowing him any space. They called round at his home day and night, without invitation, and if he didn't answer his door, they would ask his housemate to open the door and, in effect, force their way in. MJ described being intruded upon by every means possible, and this, he said, was terrifying and created such hopelessness in him that he was driven to hiding in a boiler cupboard to gain some sense of safety from his parents. This was on top of much paranoia and, therefore, vulnerability. On hearing such experiences, it is challenging to have compassion for MJ's parents. It seems that their anxieties of one son having died in such tragic circumstances and their daughter becoming estranged led to MJ being the subject of overwhelming projections, which had nothing to do with MJ's needs or human rights.

Additionally, MJ shared with me in therapy how all attempts by psychiatry for MJ to be allowed independence was met with such fierce resistance from Kenzo to the extent that Kenzo did the exact opposite of what was recommended by the psychiatrist and of which any skilled mental health practitioner would advise. MJ helped me understand that Kenzo was acting against basic healthy parenting and advocating the worst possible steps, which would only take any person into ill health. MJs only semi-safe place was to hide in the cramped boiler cupboard in his own flat, by now completely on edge at the thought of the next intrusion by his parents. MJ decided to tell his parents that he had moved to try to gain a safe space where he lived. Out of desperation, he told them that he had moved to another area and that he was working there. MJ's parents believed him, and this caused some respite for over two years, which is quite extraordinary. Akari, who started contacting MJ more, came to visit him at his home, and as they hugged for the first time in four years, he exclaimed, 'You're a bag of bones'. Akari had lost a lot of weight through her housing ordeal. It seems that MJ's parents were not able to communicate love to their children and had lost two of them for the period when Akari felt the need to estrange herself to gain a home, survival and respite.

MJ portrayed to me in therapy how he and Akari were reunited and how he had been exposed to the trauma of his mother's breast cancer. In a lonely marriage, Eml positioned herself as needing MJ, but it also became clear that Kenzo also needed MJ to stand in for him when he was absent to keep Eml company, who struggled emotionally being on her own and had fallen a few times. MJ's parents were not going to let him go. Akari noticed this and discussed her view with MJ, who was very distraught. He had taken to drinking alcohol (beer), something that Akari had been able to give up alongside tobacco and pot. Akari started visiting MJ more and was very concerned, according to MJ, about his mental health. According to MJ, she was particularly concerned that he was drinking and taking medication at the same time. One day, when she called to see him, she saw he was undressed on his stairs, and intuitively recognising his vulnerability, she gently, sensitively but firmly coaxed her brother up the stairs and instructed him quietly to put his clothes on, as if talking to a very young child, as Akari recounted to me in a one-to-one family session, from my clinical notes:

> I came to visit MJ, entered his flat and saw him sitting on his stairs naked. I immediately realized that he was not well and very vulnerable and said 'MJ let's go into the living room'. He said nothing which is unusual and entered his living room. I asked him how he was and he said nothing. I gently said to him 'Let's put some clothes on, where are your clothes?'. MJ left the room and I followed him, standing outside his bedroom door out of respect and not to evoke his possible paranoia. MJ returned with his clothes and I coaxed him gently but firmly to put on his T-shirt and I helped him with each item when needed, until he was fully dressed. I felt that I was speaking with a toddler and so acutely aware of his vulnerability. MJ then went and sat in a chair near the table, started rolling an imaginary cigarette, lit it with an imaginary lighter and smoked the cigarette, tipping the ash regularly into an imaginary ash-tray, in exactly the same place each time. Once MJ finished this cigarette, he rolled another one and continued similarly. It was quite something to behold. He didn't speak. I asked him if he realized that there was no ash-tray and he pointed to where the imaginary ash-tray was in exactly the same place as he had indicated. I was shocked but stayed with him. MJ didn't speak unless I spoke to him. I said to MJ that I was phoning the doctor since I felt afraid of what may happen next. A mental health team arrived and the CPN was aggressive. I stood up and said directly 'There is no need to talk to my brother like that, stand back, leave him alone he's in a vulnerable state'. The CPN backed off appearing full of rage. I said to the team to go, since MJ seemed understandably agitated by their presence. I waited for my dad to arrive and we all went in the car to the hospital.

I (author) was on the ward when MJ was admitted; I usually speak to new admissions onto the ward. By this time, Akari had left the hospital:

> We sat in the family room, MJ, his father and me. I sat next to MJ and his father on the other side of the table. MJ appeared separate from everyone, detached. He didn't look at anyone or seem to notice if anyone took notice of him. I observed MJ take the imaginary cigarette papers from his right hand pocket and lay them on the table, then taking one out of the packet. He lay the paper between two fingers on his right hand and opened a packet of tobacco with the other and pulled some out and lay it across the paper. MJ then rolled the imaginary cigarette, putting a filter between his lips and then inserting this at one end of the

cigarette. MJ shook the cigarette to even out the amount and placed it in his mouth. He took an imaginary lighter from his pocket and flicked this on and lit the imaginary rolled cigarette in the exact timing that it would normally take to do so. He then smoked the cigarette taking it from his mouth and blowing out what would be smoke. He flicked the ash in an imaginary ashtray on the table and continued smoking, finding the exact place as before for the ashtray every time. He even yelped at the cigarette getting too small and burning his finger, sat at the table and started rolling an imaginary cigarette, which he did with great care. He then lit it with a lighter and as he smoked it he tipped the ash in an imaginary ashtray in exactly the same place each time. Once MJ had snuffed the cigarette out he started rolling another one and repeated this numerous times, much to my interest. I wondered if MJ was displaying either delirium tremens or a form of psychosis. We waited for 20 minutes and then I called the mental health team again. I sought MJ's permission first, he looked at me and nodded and I considered that although he likely did not demonstrate having capacity, the intervention was in relation to maintaining the trust between them and upholding respect to help MJ feel safe in such a vulnerable circumstance. The mental health team arrived and I think quite aggressively, far from what was needed with this man in such a regressed state. I beckoned the mental health team to leave and went outside briefly to speak with them, regarding the sensitivity of this situation, which seemed to have escaped them, as if they had not adjusted from the ward to this vulnerable human being. When the team reentered the room where MJ sat smoking, they had calmed down. The staff assessed his mental state and he could not answer most of the everyday questions about time, place, political leader etc. and decided to detain him for his own safety. The observations and further assessment with the doctor the next day, concluded that MJ had been suffering with delirium tremens as withdrawal from alcohol, and he was discharged back to his home after one night. During the next day, I met with MJ one to one and he seemed a lot more contained in himself, not smoking the imaginary cigarettes any longer but I wondered about what he was communicating about addiction and obsessionally. He talked about his parents not leaving him alone and that he was in a gay relationship. It seemed that his personal and social boundaries were being violated from several people, trying to find respite or self-soothing through alcohol and smoking, both oral gratifications.

I reflected on how MJ's exactly repetitive actions, such as rolling and smoking cigarettes and tipping the ash in the ashtray in exactly the same spot each time, led me to consider this as a possible display of obsessive compulsivity. He denies recalling the rolling and smoking of cigarettes experience at all. Yet memory is a significant theme regarding MJ since he talks about feeling blank, and I am unsure if this is a reasonably considered side effect of the clozapine that he was started on many years ago. His short-term memory seems fine, but his long-term memory is not unreliable but absent, which concerned me. There appeared to be an investment, at least from MJ's father, in diagnosing MJ with paranoid schizophrenia and later attributing his seizures to epilepsy, despite MJ's father having no medical training. I wondered about what this may be about. MJ certainly appeared to have had psychotic episodes in thinking that he was being moved out of the country.

MJ recounted in therapy how Kenzo had responded when Kaito, MJ's brother, had died tragically and he and Akari needed to see his body to come to terms with believing his death. Kenzo was deeply opposed to them going to the chapel of peace, but together, they stood their ground, believing this to be essentially important to them. Kenzo called in a psychiatrist and a social worker to try to persuade MJ and Akari not to go ahead with this. However, the psychiatrist explored with Kenzo what this meant to him, and it transpired that Kenzo was experiencing very distressing flashbacks to when his mother had died of cancer. This helped Akari and MJ to be able to visit the chapel of peace and served as an essential aspect of grieving for both of them to date.

As a trained and qualified psychotherapist who has undergone a full personal analysis and additional personal therapy over many years, I admit to finding MJ's life extremely painful and rage-evoking in my countertransference. It seems that the expression of anger is prohibited and medicated out of existence, not only by Kenzo, who seems to communicate the rules in the family home, but also due to the impossibility of being able to express aggression and anger to Eml, who presents as emotionally fragile and vulnerable in terms of her confidence and self-esteem. In many individuals, this creates a self-referencing feedback loop, where rather than experiencing the caregiver's help, the child digests the feelings; the child is required to suppress difficult feelings to save the mother's life. It is very distressing for a child to feel angry but not be able to express this due to physical and mental ill health, at times resulting in various forms of self-harm.

In therapy, MJ shared with me about how he had been sent to a homeless hostel and how this was badly staffed with a very unclean environment, such as finding the kitchen unusable, spending this time chatting with others in the unit, watching TV, shopping out and about or sleeping. He attended some groups. MJ was also a prolific jazz drummer and pianist, having played in bands at public events. It seemed that at this time, MJ's parents wished to travel and him being in this accommodation allowed them to do so. He started having non-epileptic seizures in this hostel, possibly due to self-neglect and a lack of proper care shown towards him and/or that his clozapine medication brought with it such debilitating side effects in relation to non-epileptic/ epileptic seizures. Following a break from therapy, MJ was seeing his male partner, who became extremely aggressive towards others in public – stating on public transport that Asian and black people needed to go home – which understandably evoked strong responses in others, usually resulting in fights and contact with the police. It was surprising that MJ, a gentle but astute soul, found himself with this man, who was aggressive towards his own ethnicity.

My own reflections were that I couldn't help being reminded from somewhere that MJ was seeking attention from his father, but he was unable or unwilling to give it and that this relationship sought reparation, or re-parenting. Sadly, MJ's parents struck up what appeared to be a respite rota, which MJ was not aware of, where his partner and MJ's parents would arrange for MJ to be with him or them. This arrangement was again reminiscent of the way Kenzo tended to cart people about, almost like nonhuman objects, not really involving their consent but meeting Kenzo's needs, to read a book/newspaper.

MJ shared with me in therapy how he and Akari had agreed together to give up alcohol and tobacco to save their lives. Akari had painfully witnessed MJ drinking through one beer bottle after another, whilst on medication, 'like a robot'. Kenzo's brother, Haruto, was likely alcoholic, and alcohol was used as a currency in the family, perhaps as a controlling mechanism, – keeping members impaired. Haruto had encouraged Akari, Kaito and MJ to drink wine with him late at night, but Eml had said not to, which they complied with, but Haruto was lonely and persistent. Haruto appeared to have timed everything immaculately, envious of Kenzo's family life; it appears he had ulterior motives to destroy it. Haruto's motto was 'Make sure, there is someone worse off than yourself'.

In weekly private therapy with me, MJ attended at the consulting room in a taxi, paid for by the government due to his having developed non-epileptic seizures, which MJ described arising out of the blue. He recounted such experiences as 'horrendous'. MJ was now an outpatient living with his parents, with whom he vowed he would only stay for six months to avoid getting involved in their business. Unfortunately, Eml and Kenzo appeared at such a low ebb in their marriage at this point, blaming each other for their son's death, having lost many friends because of this. MJ, at his lowest point of having broken his ankle in the psychosis unit, was forced to live with them. At least, in their home, he would have a bed and food. When he broke his ankle, the unit manager persuaded him to go to the hospital with his sister, Akari, so that the manager would not have to complete the paperwork. The lack of care in the psychosis unit sounded concerning. The cold self-interest of this staff member towards an extremely vulnerable person was frightening. What else was occurring?

MJ shared with me in therapy how he had been suffering from non-epileptic seizures since visiting his male partner, 'Mick', who lived far from his parents. MJ recounted blacking out on the toilet and falling, requiring hospitalisation. Mick wouldn't allow any of MJ's family near him and caused arguments on the ward, to the extent that the nurse in charge had to ask him to leave. It seemed that Mick felt so acutely vulnerable when his relationship with MJ was threatened, or when Mick was on public transport, that he acted out aggressively, picking fights with people of colour. Mick lived in a dark, unfurnished flat, with his brother and their friend, who was alcoholic. MJ seemed to have found a way to separate from his parents through Mick. Their relationship lasted ten years, going on numerous holidays around the UK. Akari was the first to refuse to be in Mick's company after she overheard Mick shouting at MJ demanding why he would not answer his phone. Mick felt entitled to turn up at MJ's unit whenever he liked in the past, raising serious concerns about their relationship. MJ had to raise a safeguarding concern about Mick's contact with MJ, when he finally decided he had to say goodbye to him since he would not stop contacting him.

Having considered MJ's situation in two separate psychoanalytic supervision settings, followed by reflection, I made a possible link with MJ between the non-epileptic seizures and parting from the distressing relationship with Mick. I was aware that MJ had experienced what appeared to be dissociative seizures when visiting Mick at his flat several years prior to MJ deciding to end the relationship. I wondered if the separation from Mick reflected the painful and sudden parting from his brother, Kaito. Whereas Kaito had left MJ and his family, in this circumstance, MJ decided upon the ending with Mick. I continued to assess what the full picture was for MJ, of what has happened in the past. From the start, I was intuitively never concerned about violence in the consulting room with MJ. I have never heard of any acts of violence involving MJ, but I remain concerned about what happens to his anger and rage, which would be a normal reaction to his circumstances, past and present. I was aware that paranoid people can appear well. I spoke with MJ about his seizures being like a bodily equivalent that happens in his mind. MJ's seizures could be considered as an encapsulated psychotic part of his personality. I continued to explore with MJ whether his seizures were linked to anything disturbing.

I was very cautious navigating where and how we went in therapy with MJ, as highlighted in supervision. As the therapy progressed, MJ had an increasing capacity to gain insight and awareness about his psychological problems. I focused on gaining understanding of what MJ may be experiencing at any point in time as part of our collaborative working relationship. I didn't feel frightened of MJ. I brought in grounding exercises almost in every session since dissociated feelings may easily distance him from awareness of the need to be grounded to function in relation to self-protection and meeting his need, which appeared almost absent to him. Grounding also helped him to clarify how his parents appeared indicated in his problems and to establish and strengthen his ability to control this own mind, rather than his mind be controlled by his parents. One supervisor was questioning MJ's diagnosis of paranoid schizophrenia and wondering how it was relevant now, as well as wondering what hearing voices meant. I had thought a lot about what hearing voices meant and explored this with MJ, who considered that his hearing voices were currently like exaggerated or louder thoughts or dialogues in his mind, which he found containing. Otherwise, MJ would not talk about it, which I respected.

I further wondered with MJ how he was moving in and out of different states of mind and how this can be understood psychodynamically or psychoanalytically. MJ and I held fruitful discussions about what the anxiety may be caused by in relation to the seizures, which took some time to allow these matters to emerge. MJ was thoughtful about this and stated that he was worried by several factors: the way his parents argued with one another, how his sister's life was progressing in contrast to his, Kenzo's unpredictability, mood swings and demotivating attitude, Kenzo disallowing MJ to do anything for himself with no choice but to insist on doing everything, his brother's sudden death, parting from Mick (male ex-partner) and the future. I held in mind that MJ was the youngest offspring, remaining at home one way or another – giving his parents a hard time, like his elder brother before he died. I think that anger being disallowed in the family as instructed by Kenzo meant that negative feelings had to be repressed, but over time, this became too much. The repressed anger resurfaced, and the only unconsciously acceptable form of outlet for Kenzo and Eml was through non-epileptic seizures, with no seeming tracking to their behaviour. It may be that such repressed feelings gave the psychiatrists and Akari a run around (Diamond, 2020).

I considered Diamond's thinking and agree that psychoanalysis is frequently appropriate regarding treating trauma, alongside holding in mind its companion, the psyche/soma – dissociation, which can interfere considerably with symbolic functioning and with associative linking. Freud had originally considered such topics, such that 'repression replaced rather than supplemented dissociation' (Diamond, 2020) as the first defensive response in relation to complex trauma. It seems imperative in order to understand the triadic nature of trauma, entailing economic or drive, structural conflict and deficit and object-relational factors. Diamond (2020) advocates for an improved treatment model, incorporating defensive dissociation in the here and now, where primary and secondary dissociation are distinguished, with these differentiated from splitting and repression. He advocates for therapeutic interventions to examine unconscious, repressed phantasies associated with the 'trauma', object-relational patterns interfering with linking and psycho-economic matters that have disrupted ego functioning, which appear very helpful guidelines (Diamond, 2020).

Whatever MJ's issues mean in relation to epilepsy or drug addiction, a core issue was of wanting me to take him on when he is such a difficult case and perhaps MJ's possible satisfaction of being a difficult case for everyone. The difficulty seems to be the expression of difficult feelings and the extent to which these were unwelcome in the family. MJ would have powerful feelings about his life and the lack of parental guidance and anxieties surrounding a tragic death in the family. One supervisor considered how MJ enjoyed being difficult and that the reason behind MJ's presentation was slightly seductive, attracting people to look after him, where he is the one in charge in ways that are not as respectful as it seems. For example, he is invited to spend a week on a brain injury ward to investigate his seizures, but before the results were issued with next steps to be discussed, MJ discharged himself, as if he doesn't want his seizures to be taken away, which are his means of significantly controlling others – his family, the medical professions and emergency services. Approximately every three weeks, MJ experienced a non-epileptic seizure that sometimes lasted up to three hours before his parents called 999 for an ambulance. Paramedics would arrive within minutes, and MJ taken by ambulance to a hospital. Usually, Kenzo would follow the ambulance and wait with MJ to be seen for a brain scan, often leaving at 3–4 AM, or MJ would be retained for monitoring. I noticed what a long time had elapsed without MJ receiving psychological input. I reflected on my own psychological profession and my bias, yet it seemed that there was some kind of parental investment in maintaining MJ's condition. On speaking with Akari, she found it very difficult to witness the ongoing suffering expressed through MJ's seizures, the waste of his life and negative impact on him and the avoidance of addressing the painful issues in the family, which MJ, perhaps, became a channel for.

I monitored MJ's seizures and linked involuntary bodily movements to possible emotional happenings in the sessions. For example, MJ considered his father to be controlling and felt that he had no choice, perhaps like a baby, which I brought into the therapeutic relationship. I thought about how a baby needs to be accompanied all of the time and how MJ puts people in this position, of tending after him 24/7. His seizures gain him a lot of attention, intruding in and taking over family life and the time of the medical staff. Perhaps, having seizures was the only way that MJ could gain physical attention from his father, who reportedly otherwise hardly spoke to MJ from behind his newspaper. Seizures are not part of the brain makeup but a condition from feelings and unconscious emotion breaking out. I spoke explicitly with MJ about what is unconscious and conscious in him. MJ, like other patients with non-epileptic seizures, find this difficult to accept and tend to think that others are doing these things to them. The gains of non-epileptic seizures for the brain lead to unconscious repetitions. Not once did MJ report anything showing on his brain scans post–non-epileptic seizures. It seems that MJ's non-epileptic seizures reflect a process occurring in his mind, where the tremor doesn't leave the family. Kenzo appeared to have PTSD symptoms, and the family and the cat all seemed to shake.

I found that MJ places me in a position of a double-bind; for example, I got him out from the taxi and into the room, much like a nanny, and I reflected on the relational impact, which I talked with MJ about. I spoke of the unconscious motives which drive what he does, including the seizure state of mind. I wondered with him, 'What is it that drives this?' I considered that MJ needs to think about the question of why it happens when it does. It is anxiety that comes to see me in the transference. What is it that makes it such a worrying experience for MJ to come and see me? I wanted to help him in his helpless-ness – getting out of the taxi, finding the therapy room. He was dependent on someone, somewhere. His engagement is with people, where they will help him in his helplessness – the baby part of him. MJ does not like this aspect of him; his parents have to look after him. Yet he seems to insist on it.

I introduced the idea of what is underneath what is going on. Perhaps MJ is caught up in the conflict of being a baby, who is parented but also wishes to be a baby. How much could he accept a wish to live like a baby? The uncon-scious wish makes him do the things – the roles that he wants to embody. MJ seems powerful in being powerless. The more helpless he is, the closer he can be to his mother. I picked up on what may be going on in his unconscious and interpreted the conflict. What if he is to make his own decisions? Currently, MJ seems to be living life like a baby, with no separation from his mother, and this is reflected in his psychological and bodily state. I challenged that the seizures undermine his confidence but that perhaps he insists on being a baby – to face the conflict where the gain is unconscious. I surmised that MJ's paranoid structure is his father's doing – a conflict with others rather than with himself. MJ seemed to have given up life for a return to babyhood. Perhaps as Klein observes, MJ was making reparation.

From therapy, it came back to me that MJ had a need to find a way to be close to his father, and the seizures offered the opportunity for this, which perhaps was sexualised. It was after MJ had parted from Mick that MJ started to spend more time with his father, albeit in a hospitalised setting. My aim was to help MJ gain understanding about his experiences, hoping that my perception may be useful to him since few may grasp his experiences. The feelings that MJ induces in others appear as enactments rather than as verbal expressions, and I focused on his sense of responsibility in these. Addition-ally, I enquired with MJ about his experiences prior to the seizure and his feelings at that time in a detailed way. For example, 'What were you doing?' 'Who was there?' and 'What was going through your mind?' I was aware that what was going through his mind may not have been in his awareness at the time of the seizure.

In supervision, we considered a sense of manic feeling, where there was something belittling occurring because others would know what to do, whereas others do not know what to do and feel powerless and perplexed. MJ's unconscious seemed to be playing with others – the toddler? Behind MJ's well-dressed and well-mannered appearance is an aim to show that he is not worth anything. MJ managed to get doctors, paramedics, family and members of the public to help him – indicating how he handles people who attempt to help him. MJ in later therapy sessions entered the consulting room hum-ming or singing, which I would acknowledge which tune he was drawing my attention to, to bring him to our relationship. MJ spoke about wanting a 'fruit-ful' relationship, which I was interested to explore what this meant to him. I wondered what kind of fruitfulness he wanted in his life. I considered that he knows how to play people. Is there something he wants to dedicate his life to? MJ was a musician and shrewd to the mundanities of nine-to-five work. Perhaps there was an issue of trust with me: one part of MJ staying where he is producing symptoms that gain help, another part that wants to do something. I wondered, 'How can he confront this sort of conflict, or how much of him wants to confront the conflict?' I considered this an issue of strategy for interpretation, and whether I could see through it and still want to continue seeing him was perhaps another issue for him.

MJ shared with me in therapy that he had gone to live on his own, away from his parents' knowledge of his whereabouts, dealing with his sexuality at the time. I was cautious about the relationship between MJ and me, given the gender difference. I pondered whether there was an uncertain identity with MJ regarding sexuality and perhaps other aspects of being male and a man – Kenzo's identity being described by MJ as 'like shifting sands' and by Eml as 'a strange personality'. MJ shared with me that he had a lot to talk about, and I explored with him what this was – sexuality or what this is about. I wondered what it meant to his mother to get married since she appeared to reject Kenzo and prioritised her children, perhaps very difficult for her to let go of her youngest, MJ, who is 'asked' to remain an infant. This may be a fundamental grievance for MJ, playing games with helpers, as a replaying of an early relationship with his mother. I reflected on this being an infantile game of resentment, where he is rejected at the moment of most need and is confused about how to be open and available. Therefore, MJ is unsure of why I want to see him, perhaps, replaying his relationship with his overanxious mother.

I am naturally curious about MJ's unconscious, keeping questions open in my mind regarding where conscious thoughts come from, with different meanings in different contexts. I recall that Freud asked questions, but I wonder what I am getting into by asking questions. Am I acting out something with the patient? I decide to keep questions to myself – an enquiry into my own experience – and when appropriate, I think about how to interpret that transference relationship, as signposts into the unconscious. However, the unconscious can be too unbearable and painful, and the question is how much of it can be revealed in psychosis, where strengthening the ego is needed, while being cautious about stirring the pot too deeply.

MJ managed to share with me that his non-epileptic seizures had taken control of his body for up to six hours a time in the psychosis unit, and because he was unable to use his phone at these times, he could not call for help in the office due to his whole body shaking. One Christmas, MJ ended up sitting on a bench as he walked out into the snow, when a seizure took form. He got stuck on the bench, frozen and unable to use his mobile phone to call for help. A couple passing by noticed his strife, but MJ stated that he was okay. MJ had not returned home, and the police eventually found him on the same bench hours later, extremely cold and frightened, stuck.

The seizures, involving severe shaking of his arms and legs, would, at times, throw MJ across the room. He would suffer head and other injuries, often breaking his skin, causing severe wounds, such as a dislocated ankle, cut forehead, bruised eyes or broken nose. MJ's insight was that these non-epileptic attacks (NEA disorder) started when he commenced clozapine. Through these NEAD seizures, MJ was able to hold a fully logical conversation, showing awareness of self and other. The first time that he returned to therapy with me from a break of a few months, he tripped as he went up the stairs to my consulting room and injured his head but picked himself up and entered the therapy room to then have a full-bodied seizure, which lasted around two hours. The seizure took him over the agreed 50 minutes of the therapy session, but I contracted with MJ to remain in the consulting room, firstly, due to concern for MJ's vulnerability. How would he get home in this state of mind? And secondly, he would learn that I could tolerate his seizures and wanted to stay and help him through this disturbing experience, as recorded in my clinical notes:

> Towards the end of this first therapy session after a few months break, MJ sat on the couch. I observed MJ having jerking movements through his arms and legs, letting out a sound as if trying to manage himself but also facially shocked by the involuntary movements. I felt perturbed and had never witnessed a non-epileptic seizure before, only what was referred to as a pseudo-seizure (fainting) observed on an acute ward in London. It was clear that this patient needed attention communicated through the seizure which appeared dissociative since MJ spoke to me completely rationally, whilst his body was out of control. I could tolerate MJ becoming dissociative alongside thinking how to help him out of this state. I suggested grounding techniques to bring him into his current situation. It was difficult for these to be managed with the extent of bodily movements. I focused on his body and his experience in the room, what he could hear, smell, taste and touch. Over 15 minutes or so, MJ's bodily movements decreased. Pacing my interventions sensitively, although MJ stated he wanted to keep talking, I endeavored to explore possible triggers for MJ's non-epileptic seizures but understood that patients often have no awareness of this. MJ at first could not think of anything but was keen to explore further, and thoughts about his sister visiting and his relationship with his mother came to mind and father being cruel to his mother. It seemed that MJ felt protective of his mother but also that she seemed to offer a relationship to MJ which could not be fulfilled, perhaps unconsciously seductively, due to her lonely and unfulfilled marriage and her need for company and support which was more considered and sensitive towards her. I observed MJ shaking on the couch for two or so hours, holding at the same time an interesting and perfectly logical conversation. My instinct was to remain still, calm

and empathic. I asked MJ what would help and he said for me to stay with him, that his parents would leave the room when this happened at the family home or they would start arguing. My intuition was to offer MJ food, although this was outside of any usual therapy boundaries. I had a box of chocolates still unfinished from Christmas and offered these to him. He ate hungrily and the sugar seemed to help him in relation to reducing his symptoms of his shaking. Perhaps, I reflected I wanted his shaking to stop, there was something unbearable about it. MJ's mind was saying one thing – I am logical and in control and his body something else. I was struck by the depth of sadness I felt, his isolation and abandonment with this situation. MJ and I discussed what he thought was going on in his body and he said that he didn't know. It was easy for me to think that this was clearly a communication of distress and trauma. I reflected what was being touched on in me, as MJ thanked me again for sitting with him. After around two hours of talking, MJ's abrupt jerking movements subsided and I talked with him about the prospect of calling a taxi, which I supported him to do and walked with him down in the lift when I noticed that MJ walked as if on the moon (dissociated) and I ensured that he was safely in the car and that MJ had communicated the address he wanted to go to the taxi driver. MJ texted me to let me know he had arrived safely at his parents' home, very unlike the usual boundaries of a therapy session. I wondered about his unmet infantile needs.

In therapy, I tried to help MJ become aware of what makes him dissociate rather than to dissociate and to bring him back into the room. I felt that there was a developing co-dependency between MJ and his mother and spoke over time about how MJ had stated that he would move back with his parents for a short time. I listened closely to MJ and learned that Kenzo needed MJ in the home as much as Eml did but that this did not meet MJ's growth and development as a person. I discussed, therefore, with MJ about him leaving home, perhaps a repeat of the adolescent phase which certainly didn't seem thought about or supported by Kenzo and Eml for their own needs. It seemed that MJ was crying out for help with this but that it was not in his parents' interests to hear and act on this developmental need. They seemed invested in MJ becoming more dependent on them and more disabled (such as leaving him to sleep until 3 PM for their own space, not providing a private space where MJ could be, controlling his medical appointments and money and MJ providing companionship to Eml as her husband slept).

In future therapy sessions, I encouraged MJ to go out more since he stayed in fearing a seizure, but once he went out, he discovered that strangers were concerned and caring towards him. He spent numerous hours in hospitals having brain scans, which never showed anything. He was called to stay on a brain injury ward for a week, where the medical team considered that he suffered from trauma. MJ's seizures attracted much attention to him, and he calmed quickly in a hospital setting away from his parents' home, which he said was relevant. His parents were nasty to each other, and he found this distressing. I considered that MJ was dependent on his parents, which was hindering his development further. Kenzo was able to watch TV politics, read his newspaper and talk with Eml, whilst MJ wasted his life, almost allocated to sleep, staying up late to have the house to himself but with no routine, purpose or structure in his life.

In subsequent therapy sessions, there was a depth of trust between MJ and I, based, I think, on him knowing that I would stay with him through emotional turmoil and that I could manage such situations. MJ reflected on the possible triggers as advised in supervision, and this approach revealed further information in relation to non-epileptic seizures at his family home. It seemed that Eml was positioning herself as almost as a surrogate wife to MJ, which also benefited Kenzo but caused bloody conflicts between them nonetheless. In therapy, MJ shared how, when his sister, Akari, was due to attend at the psychosis unit, he had dislocated and broken his ankle, and similarly, he had a seizure when Akari visited the parental home. I recognised that there was a lot of annoyance around in relation to the seizures. I wondered if he felt pressured to communicate about matters that he found difficult to put into words – his communication being, like his mother, largely non-verbal.

MJ shared with me in therapy that he had completed a degree at an elite university and, therefore, had inner resources but that he had not kept up his skills since then. Perhaps they would be easily revived. MJ would talk in detail and engagingly about science. It seems that there was difficulty in knowing who he is. MJ spoke about fears and delusions of being invaded and taken over, with no seeming private space in his home or personality either. It was difficult to feel that he has his own life and personality, and I talked to him about this in subsequent sessions. I wondered with MJ about what it means to have his own life, space and boundary. MJ had attempted this in the past, but he reported his parents taking over his flat space, which was distressing. I talked with MJ about what he considered were the aims of therapy. I wondered if he came to therapy to be in touch with his strength. MJ felt that the therapy is a space to think about his feelings, without abuse from his parents and partner. I spoke with MJ that he can rely on the therapy space not to be a bullying space, that it is not an abusive space. I wondered what the nature of the abuse from his partner was. MJ spoke about feeling very paranoid about the phone calls between his parents and his partner, as they arranged MJ's care without consultation with him. He felt that Mick (partner), his brother and friend were ganging up on him and taking his money when he was asleep (through clozapine and other medications).

MJ managed to share with me in therapy that his body was very frightened and felt abused in the non-epileptic seizure, which he reported had lasted for four hours. He was finding a space that he can trust, something he had never had before with his parents and partner but imagined he could have with his sister. Gradually, MJ was becoming able to talk about things, including abuse from his male partner, in a space he can trust. I envisaged that MJ could look at all the moments in his life, considering which space is he in at any particular moment, in case he is in danger. His life is so unstable that he might be safe or unsafe, which appeared to be a critical issue all day, every day. MJ may appear compliant and may feel that his relationship with psychiatry is unsafe at times. MJ appeared to have given up on life, remaining on benefits. I spoke with MJ about his life appearing to be divided into two spaces: trustworthy and bullying. I considered a possible connection between judgement, bullying and trust, linked to the non-epileptic seizures. However trustworthy, the space will become dubious for him – from time to time, a bullying space, at others, a threatening space. The trusted space becomes dangerous, and I can become dangerous and bullying. It seems that reality is not a steady thing in psychosis. I thought that I will become a bullying object, having to comply with me to avoid the abuse from me in the transference. When discussing confidentiality, MJ showed a deep suspicion of me that I was creeping into the space he was trying to keep pure and trustworthy. In psychoanalysis, the task of therapy is to recognise that no space is completely good or bad and to make the most of the space he has in therapy.

In therapy, I worked hard to create a situation that was safe enough for him to bring his feelings. Psychoanalytically, I took up his sudden fears that I was doing awful things to him. I noticed the moment when the safe space threatened to change, where I abused his boundaries and he had to work hard to bring it back to the prior situation of being eternally trustworthy. I noticed that I was making a great deal of effort to keep it trustworthy and to keep it pure. Much of the work felt like there was an intellectual understanding by MJ but also an emotional transference that I was perfectly trustworthy, and MJ was moved and overwhelmed at having a perfect therapist who listened to him with perfect accuracy. MJ needs this idealised image, then he can be happy, but the longer it goes on, the more wobbly it will become. MJ appeared to comply to avoid abuse. I tried to help MJ understand the process of therapy and repeated the importance of confidentiality to help him feel safe in each session. I also explained that there might be exceptions and discussed this to enable him to feel in control. I would discuss any third-party contact with him first, including what would be said with his input and consent, and there would be a follow-up conversation with him after any such external contact, which would be in exceptional circumstances. I acknowledged that a plethora of feelings were around and moved away from conflict by spelling out more concretely what I understood to be occurring.

MJ shared with me in therapy how, on his birthday, he experienced multiple seizures, and together, we sought to understand the triggers. For example, a seizure started after 'Happy Birthday' was sung on his birthday. I spoke with him about whether he was getting close to having a seizure and if he can talk about it without having another seizure. I sought to help him recognise a danger signal prior to a seizure. Likewise, I discussed with him what the triggers were prior to a seizure in the particular instant that it happened. Additionally, I was interested in what his feelings were when people were singing 'Happy Birthday'. MJ is not in a position of control when under seizure, and I focused on centring him through breathing and distracting him into the present. I applied grounding techniques, such as having him feel the bounds of his arms and legs, stomping his feet to feel the pressure and, when he was less aroused, checking whether he is with me. From the start of the sessions, I centred him to help him being overly aroused. I considered the dissociated affect from MJ's conscious mind expressed through his body.

Upon personal reflection, I realised what a huge emotional factor it is who MJ talks to about what, given his seeming little control over his life and his parents' skewed boundaries. I had wondered what the emotional feeling to his birth was. What does it mean to MJ to be getting older? The paramedics regularly attend to his seizures (on average, once every three weeks) but not the huge emotional problem. I acknowledged that I thought that he was avoiding something and posed that if it was intolerable, why not avoid it? MJ would often leave the therapy session shaking, and his vulnerability is very saddening for me. I wondered about this transferentially, especially in relation to his mother and what MJ was possibly communicating to me unconsciously and 'asking' me to hold and digest. Supervision with Dr. Duncan McLean advised being more straight with MJ. It was true that I felt hesitant to trigger his seizures, but I learned that gentle and firm communication helped him. MJ recounted that our discussions about going out into the world rather than waiting at home in case a seizure occurred, led MJ to attend a jazz gig which he had not done for several years. He is a jazz musician of a range of instruments. When at the gig, he had a full non-epileptic seizure, and the kind staff at the pub called an ambulance for him, as he struggled on the floor.

I reflected on this incident with a mix of feelings emerging. MJ was surprised at how helpful members of the public were towards him, increasing his trust in the world and making him question whether he needed to be so dependent on his parents. It seemed that he desperately needed people to attend to him and make him feel cared for. Having met with his parents and sister, his father was very focused on himself almost superficially and his mother preoccupied with her own needs. MJ's need for attention became a public nuisance at the gig, and people only knew him for a short time. This gave him some attention. It is a job to recognise MJ's attention-seeking behavior, as well as to recognise attention-seeking, which is absolutely desperate and has destroyed his life. This need to be cared for has destroyed his life. MJ seems to know that it is appropriate for him to leave home, but he can't do it because his body feels seizures, an anchoral state within him, highlighting the need for extreme and permanent care and attention – like a belief system acted out through his body, where he doesn't have to be aware of what it means. I wondered if he really wanted to know about what his body is expressing. Should he be in therapy? What is he avoiding that attracts attention in a different way from how he behaves? There is an emotional factor – getting care and attention that he believes he needs, destroying his career. Something inside him says that he believes. It is different for him – a baby-like state of needing Mum and Dad to rescue him and repair his unmet needs, with them not meeting these needs in order to keep him in a baby state to fulfil their own needs. MJ, therefore, has not moved on from this properly, as if he still needs baby care and attention.

I considered that it seems that MJ is driven by a desperation, which I didn't have a picture of. I thought that MJ thought that the desperation will overwhelm him and me, and I interpreted this to him. I think that he has the resources to be an independent, functioning adult. Why is his desperation stronger than anyone else's? It may be that his parents' neglect of him has left him in a double-bind. I communicated to MJ that I can manage the desperation of need of care and attention by way of wanting to settle these things with him. I hoped that showing understanding would lead to making boundaries and assessed whether he can take the therapy. I wanted to edge towards discussing this question with MJ but not before any summer break. The answer to the question may be fury at not being given care and attention, only known through his body with seizures. Perhaps he is unconsciously furious when people don't pay attention and is desperate for it. MJ remains so dependent on people and hates them because of their being good at care and attention. He is furious if he doesn't get it – impossible. There is a conflict that he brings, which is only attended to by his body in this desperate way. I asked MJ how he feels about the break, but he didn't know. I was firm, definite and empathic. MJ sang a lot in the sessions leading to the break, perhaps a surging distraction from his experience of feeling discarded from my care. I felt the singing was rageful. I didn't interrupt the singing with a question since I felt otherwise the rage may be put into a bodily seizure. In my countertransference, I felt that the break was too much to face for MJ. I wondered if the break was too much to face with someone willing to understand, or does he want me to collude with avoidance behaviour?

I pondered on what happens to the feelings of a non-epileptic seizure. I considered that MJ was fearful about what's inside him. He appeared to be in a relationship in his mind, where one part is angry, identified as his father. This may be a part of himself – a seemingly disturbed part of himself which frightens him, who could be as raging and as destructive as he is. MJ gets very close to his mother instead. It is the disturbed part of him which leads to seizures, identified with his father. It may be too difficult to face that his father is a part of him. Perhaps MJ is like an Oedipal victor who has triumphed over the father. Kenzo (father) may be fed up with him intruding on the marital relationship, as MJ seemed locked into the primal scene. MJ shared with me about the psychosis unit, where his next-door neighbour, a nice, obese woman who smelt of urine, had her urine seep under his bedroom door. The staff were reportedly neglectful, and there appear to be two versions: one idealised (mother) and one ghastly (father), where MJ feels he is nothing. MJ's recounting of the hostel reveals these two versions of how he may be feeling with me. I was cautious not to fall into the trap that he occupies with me – the husband. I discussed the two alternative versions of who I am. I thought that behind these versions are seizures, occupying the attention of his parents exclusively. All the attention is on him; he is the centre of attention because he is so frightened of what will happen if he loses that. He feels pissed on and neglected.

Regarding MJ, I wondered which transference is operative at a particular moment. By sitting with him for two hours, I am exclusively occupied by listening to him. I considered the silences when an exclusive relationship with me gets lost, and he perhaps has to struggle to suppress another view of me – that of a psychotherapist who has two parts that he can't understand. One part of him occupies me or the mother, and another part rages about people, like the psychosis unit staff who prefer to paint their nails. It was discussed for him to move out of the home and to dare to leave his parents on their own. MJ's emotional state felt like an explosion inside him, erupting into a seizure and then being contained in the hospital, this safe area for MJ. However, at other times, MJ would not allow silence and would hum or sing. I thought that, due to the exclusionary sense of silence, he broke away and pieced together his dread of seizures, which were provoked by having to be with other people whilst his parents were left in the primal scene. I wondered what he made of the deprivation. In his mind, I reflected on my position as the husband that he is desperate to cancel out. The transference to me is that I represent the husband being killed off, which becomes the cause of the husband being absent. I thought further about MJ's possible guilt and his potential to feel guilty about something – such as killing off the brother. MJ grew to look like his brother who died, perhaps expressing a wish to find his brother resurrected in him. I wondered if MJ felt that I was pissing on him.

It was interesting for me to explore with MJ in therapy the time when Akari was due to attend the family home, but Eml had sat on MJ's bed and chatted with him. Kenzo had entered the room and could be cantankerous and possessive of Eml, expressing this by bullying her. MJ stood up for his mother to his father, and a huge argument erupted, leading to a non-epileptic seizure, involving MJ cutting his head and bruising both eyes. I wondered about how Eml was positioning herself, possibly seductively in relation to MJ but also linked with Kenzo too. It seemed that MJ was being used by both parents: by Eml for pleasant and fun company when Kenzo was either working as a trustee or asleep and by Kenzo for MJ to stand in as a surrogate husband, enabling Kenzo to do what he wanted – all for free rent. In this way, MJ perhaps became trapped due to his dependence on his parents for love, a home and financial support, as well as emotional support and companionship.

I felt saddened and thought that perhaps the only way that anger, upset, etc., could be expressed in this threesome was non-verbally, just as often distress is expressed in physical illness. I discussed MJ's confidence to move forward in his life, and he told me that he had become a carer to his parents but that was never acknowledged by them and that they refer to all the help they gave him. I told MJ to move out, but the parents needed him there to survive, and MJ believed that this was his only route to survival. Kenzo controlled what could be talked about in the family – football, politics, books but never anything personal or emotional. Although Kenzo was an emotional man, he shut this down in himself and others. Eml was extremely emotional, and tears were just under the surface, especially regarding her son Kaito, who had died tragically, and other associated losses. I was aware of MJ being in a very difficult situation. It was apparent to me that MJ needed his parents, however much they were undermining him but with little sense that he can survive on his own. This was perhaps linked with his parents' inability to help him to separate emotionally and his confidence in his ability to do so, which was deliberately undermined consistently by Kenzo and Eml. I recall feeling a powerful anger and sadness in my countertransference, thinking about how I felt that MJ's vulnerability was being taken advantage of, alongside his pull to wanting to be looked after, likely returning to an early childhood phase of unmet need, perhaps at the toddler phase, reflecting what I had observed during his delirium tremens psychosis when MJ rolled and smoked imaginary cigarettes.

I discussed with MJ in his therapy how safe he feels with me and when this is not the case. MJ repeated that he feels a sense of safety with me. We explored this sense of safety in detail. It was a collaborative process of looking at something together, and I communicated being sensitive to this in the room. In this way, MJ and I explored and clarified how robust he, in fact, is and how he feels safe. I discussed in supervision how overly careful I thought MJ was with me – perfectionistic, in the transference revealing and working through a fragile and vulnerable mother whose life he needed to save, both in a seemingly surrogate father and husband role, both of which were historically absent. It seems likely that when MJ dissociated and neared awareness, the feelings threatened to overwhelm him. I paid a lot of attention to how he entered the consulting room and what he brought with him, as if he were in an ordinary state of mind, yet what came into the room with him was something else. MJ's life was strewn with trouble for him in the way that he is functioning. I came to think that his feelings about his sister were perhaps linked to the reality of MJ's life coming to the fore when she visited, along with the associated feelings perhaps of shame, humiliation and frustration. It seemed that MJ felt depressed by his sister, who had managed to live an independent life of her own. I explored which aspects of MJ's life were functional and was very careful about how I made him feel about potential dysfunctionality to get hold of his sense of agency, constantly and persistently undermined by his parents' unmet needs, and to clarify how he would like his life to be different. I was aware that if he manages something, that's great, but if I encourage him, he may also feel bad about not being able to do it.

Interestingly, when MJ brought photographs to therapy of his family and himself, it was striking that he had come to look very similar to his elder brother, Kaito, in their physical appearances. I reflected on this and on MJ's comment that he recounted in a therapy session that 'I'm here so that Akari doesn't have to look for Kaito anywhere else', aligned with suicidality where the grieving person seeks to join their deceased loved one. It seemed that MJ had unconsciously come to look like Kaito to, in his mind, save Akari's life, just as he had been the person in the family who drew Akari back to the family when she had become estranged. MJ looking like Kaito saved his parents their grief as if Kaito lived on through MJ (Freud, 1917). MJ was unconsciously the glue in the family. The loss of their eldest son meant that they had to control MJ all the more, becoming the container of their anxious projections. He was not allowed to move and became more home-based as time went on, following a spate of long-distance walking and exploring outside. Eml and Kenzo both needed MJ to live with them to hold the marriage together. MJ became a stabiliser for them despite being the family member, presumably most fragile, with a diagnosis of paranoid schizophrenia. Yet MJ was very empathic, sociable, observant and understanding, which didn't fit with such a diagnosis. MJ, however, spoke of feeling out of reality through experiences of paranoia, which he found extremely distressing. He spoke of his memory not functioning properly, as stated earlier. When his sister tried to encourage MJ to attend therapy, he was adamant that he would not, then shared with her that he would find it too hard to face to talk about his elder brother and other experiences. MJ's non-epileptic seizures controlled the family, leading to multiple hospitalisations. Akari decided to live at a distance and found it very painful to step into the family home to be met with such immense unprocessed pain and violence. She recounted in a one-to-one session with me that, when she was at the family home at Christmas, everyone had gone out, leaving her on her own for the majority of the day. Then her father caused an argument and kicked her out in the snow. Akari shared about feeling unable to stay in the same room as her family and feeling pushed out by the raw emotion, often sitting on her own in a separate room. She spoke sadly of finding it excruciating witnessing such severe neglect of her brothers, and feeling totally powerless to change the situation, she could only feel utterly sad or become hyperactive in focusing on building her life, with ongoing guilt related to surviving her elder and younger brothers and not wanting to be like MJ or her parents.

MJ shared with me in therapy how Akari remained single to rescue her younger brother, not trusting her parents to look after him properly and actually considering the situation as abusive. She saw Freud's 'Mourning and Melancholia' paper demonstrated by MJ, who took on the identity of his elder brother to keep the need for the family to mourn at bay and to save his sister from trying to join Kaito in death. She had been close to him and placed in the role of surrogate mother, with Kaito speaking only to Akari for the last four years of his life. MJ shared that Eml hardly slept and experienced intrusive thoughts about Kaito's death, managed only through listening to the radio every night.

Now MJ appears healthy, although perhaps needing to lose weight, food perhaps being his only comfort in his parents' home, where he neither has a purpose in life nor a romantic partner, with no limits set to help him know where he starts and ends. His anti-psychotic medication could be responsible for his weight gain. He appears cognitively and emotionally well, astute, highly observant and insightful in therapy, with an appropriate sense of humour. However, the extent of his medication led me to suggest a medication review via supervision, but MJ doesn't want to do that. He remains perhaps overinvolved with his mother and entangled, therefore, within his parents' marriage. Kenzo's moods are unpredictable and nasty, alongside Eml being capable of bullying and being equally nasty. Akari feels trapped to not abandon MJ, who has few if no friends, although he is well-liked. She throws herself into being amongst normal people and trying to develop her career, only sharing with very few people about her family situation since, by association, she had experienced much prejudice and lack of understanding.

**Conclusions**

MJ had been a child with difficulties from the start, including being partially sighted, having been colic as a baby, socially phobic at school, dyslexic and the youngest in a family, where there were significant past traumas that repeated themselves. Due to Kenzo's sensitivity to being in the family, Eml had perhaps not received the emotional support needed for parenting three young children, with Kenzo working away from home. Perhaps with a lack of a father figure, MJ did not develop a strong-enough sense of self to navigate the world, and with others being envious of his capabilities, he didn't like conflict and, therefore, may have shied away from confrontation and withdrew. In his family, MJ seemed to be the glue for the family stability, with his clear insights and observations and being able to talk to his parents in ways that worked for all concerned. MJ has not only lost his brother but his sister had also been estranged for some four years, which was likely to have been very distressing for him. There appears to be a difficulty of individuating from Eml and Kenzo and a need to keep their offspring dependent. This would interfere with their growth and development. To date, MJ appears healthy-looking and is lively minded with positive cognitive health. MJ's non-epileptic seizures have reduced considerably, perhaps due to a focus on processing his past traumas, establishing and maintaining a routine, offering a safe and confidential space to share in, clarifying family dynamics and thinking with MJ about meeting his needs, which have clearly been greatly overlooked for myriad reasons.

# 6 Case study 2 – 'Jennie' – a case of deep grief

This case study intends to provide accurate descriptions and reflections of my classical person-centred and pluralistic-relational therapeutic work with Jennie on an acute female ward in London. I thought to adapt my usual psychoanalytic stance due to working on a ward, as discussed in supervision with Professor Robert Hinshelwood. The aim is to demonstrate my ability to apply psychotherapeutic theory to practice, illuminated by the reasoning that informs my clinical decisions throughout. Regarding the ten-minute excerpt of a therapeutic session, the focus will be on the process of therapy – what may be happening between the client and me, alongside critically reflecting on practice and offering a micro-level analysis of the therapeutic work. This opens up an opportunity to explore and discuss my responses to specific client exchanges, alongside management of the therapeutic relationship and alternate interventions.

## Introduction to client

'Jennie' is a retired female black-British mid-60-year-old nurse and midwife of West Indian descent. She has three children and grandchildren and lives in her home with her son. 'Jennie' separated from her children's father and subsequent partner, both alcoholic and sexually abusive. When 'Jennie's' father died, a gambler and alcoholic, she 'broke down'; her mother died in 2014. I selected this material questioning how to work with 'Jennie's' self-concept from a person-centred perspective[1].

## Context of the work

This therapeutic work took place on a psychosis unit for women aged 18–65 years. The ward has 25 beds on two corridors, with a central lounge area and TV, nursing station, doctor's and administrative offices, dining room, quiet room and activity room. The atmosphere is noisy and challenging, the TV loudly transmitting pop music, to which some women dance to, including both patients and staff. Many verbal and physical fights take place in this communal area, seemingly due to intense frustrations and, at times, lack of nursing staff present.

DOI: 10.4324/9781003509059-7

## Theoretical approach

The theoretical approach in my work with 'Jennie' is classical person-centred, informed by grief work as a process of meaning-making (Neimeyer et al., 2014), alongside work with people diagnosed with schizophrenia, as pioneered by Rogers and experientially by Gendlin, Kiesler and Truax (Rogers, 1957; Rogers et al., 1967). My interest was to explore using interventions from a different therapeutic modality to gauge whether the client benefited from it. These influences, mentioned earlier, are central to my development as a psychotherapist, although the Wisconsin project suffered due to unclear measurements. However, my prior training has been in psychoanalytic and psychodynamic interventions, but intuitively, my work with Jennie called upon the core conditions, alongside an analytic stance with a mind for unconscious dynamics.

My rationale for adopting the person-centred approach is that the conditions of worth facilitate actualisation and a range of emotion-focused interventions available for people in crisis. Pre-therapy (Van Werde & Prouty, 2007) sought to restore 'psychological contact', one of Rogers's necessary and sufficient conditions (Rogers, 1957, 1959) for reciprocal relationships alongside the seven stages of process change (Rogers, 1961a). Pre-therapy was adapted by me for one client on the ward without relevance to 'Jennie'. Additional contemporary counselling and psychological approaches that are invaluable to my role are, for example, psychotherapy activity preferences (Cooper et al., 2021); identity incongruent discrimination (Franco et al., 2021); Covid-19 guidance (British Psychological Society, 2021; Laslo-Roth et al., 2021); and strength-oriented practice (Bartholomew et al., 2020). No psychometric measures were employed.

The philosophical antecedents of the person-centred approach to therapy are humanism, existentialism and phenomenology. There are additional relational-ethical (Gilligan, 1982) and pluralistic influences (Mearns & Cooper, 2018), which I critique. Ethically, I wonder about responsibility becoming blurred with focus on the betweenness of therapist and client, where responsibility can conceivably be avoided. My person-centred approach involved clearing a safe one-to-one space and offering my psychologically holding presence nurtured through psychoanalysis (Elliott & Westwell, 2012), alongside interventions based on the following core conditions: congruence, unconditional positive regard and empathy (Rogers, 1957) with agreed goals (Cooper & Law, 2018) and preferences (Cooper & Norcross, 2021). Goal-setting is arguably a directive practice but supports the direction of actualising. Interestingly, Jennie did not want to set any goals initially.

## Referral information

The client self-referred for therapy with me, in consultation with the multi-disciplinary team. The presenting issue was the loss of 'Jennie's' father.

## Assessment

'Jennie' approached me on the ward for therapy, whilst grieving her father's death. Having introduced myself to 'Jennie' as a therapist, the contractual terms were discussed in relation to the following: confidentiality with exceptions of harm to self or other and my person-centred therapeutic approach comprising weekly open-ended sessions. Additionally, Jennie's understanding was checked, alongside informing her of the complaint process. 'Jennie's' mental capacity to consent was assessed regarding her understanding, retention, weighing up and communication of information. Accessible language was used to explain that the audio-recorded sessions were for use in supervision/professional practice seminars, where recorded and written material from 'Jennie's' sessions, including transcribed extracts, may also be used for publication by me. Records of sessions would be stored in accordance with General Data Protection Regulation (Data Protection Act, 2020). 'Jennie' was given time to consider this request alongside my answering any questions she may have. 'Jennie' signed the service user consent form, which was then stored in a locked cabinet, only accessible by myself. Jennie was eager for our work to be shared with as many as possible, since she felt that it may help others which was very generous of her, but I further reflected about this regarding safeguarding her.

'Jennie' was well-presented with a large build, holding consistent eye contact with me. She appeared intelligent, talkative but guarded, distressed and assertive. Jennie's disinhibited talking appeared to distance others. 'Jennie' shared how, as a toddler, her poverty-stricken family migrated from the West Indies to London during the Windrush. The eldest of six siblings, 'Jennie' was a child-carer, her father an alcoholic gambler, leading to further poverty.

'Jennie' married a sexually abusive alcoholic man, then they separated. Albeit hard, 'Jennie' enjoyed mothering her two daughters and son. Regarding her career as a nurse and midwife, 'Jennie' expressed pride. 'Jennie' reported blocking a recent alcoholic partner, alongside her son giving him access to her home, alerting safeguarding issues, with a social worker being involved.

Jennie's mother died, and when Jennie 'broke down', she then nursed her father, who had cancer and died in 2019, at which point Jennie 'broke down' again. She said, 'Witnessing his drinking broke my heart'. Jennie's close uncle died later. Jennie conveyed witnessing her parents experiencing racism in the '50s and '60s, describing her father as 'Indian and English'. Jennie identified as a Black Lives Matter activist, wanting racial harmony in juxtaposition to family conflicts.

Jennie was admitted to a hospital by ambulance. A neighbour observed Jennie absconding through an upper-storey window, reportedly locked in by her son. In December, Jennie was discharged for home treatment.

Two weeks later, she was being readmitted by her son, under Section 2 of the Mental Health Act (1983).[2] Since Jennie attended the weekly therapy group that I facilitate on the ward, we discussed the boundaries around the two contexts, alongside the impact on our therapeutic relationship. In the group, I assessed Jennie's interpersonal skills. Jennie dominated the space without apparent awareness of others, seeking company yet intolerant of opinions differing from hers, with childlike tantrums ensuing.

## Formulation

According to the British Psychological Society *Practice Guidelines* (2011), formulation is a summary of the integration of the knowledge obtained through the assessment process, drawing on psychological theory and research to offer a framework for summarising the client's needs (British Psychological Society, 2017, p. 10). This case formulation is considered a humanistic collaborative discussion, prioritising client choice, autonomy and their expertness by experience (Simms, 2011, p. 24). Formulation is arguably incompatible with person-centred practice when therapist-directed (Rogers, 1951). However, clients express finding a collaboratively formed summary of their needs helpful.

A formulation based on Simms's model (2011) follows conceptualising the client's conflicts in person-centred terms. The conditions of worth (Rogers, 1957) laid down in Jennie's childhood appear genderised and racialised (Chantler, 2005): emotional neglect and abuse, child-parenting, racial exposure and paternal addiction, leading to incongruence, conditional regard and judgement. Jennie's introjected values and beliefs appear fear-based. Jennie's self-concept is based on paying for validation and taking responsibility to gain control. Additionally, Jennie expressed feeling abandoned, sad and lonely, her self-concept possibly affected due to her race, alongside possibly internalising racial oppression. Aspects of denial and distortion of experience were present through Jennie feeling unworthy of love and deserving of abusive partners. Jennie wants society to be one harmonious family. Her favourite song, *One Love/People Get Ready* (Marley & The Wailers, 1977) painfully contrasts her family situation. Jennie gives her money away, leaving herself poorer, perhaps not considering herself as enough.

These experiences present a state of incongruence; despite 'Jennie's' professional and family achievements, she feels abandoned, particularly through Covid-19. Regarding the actualising tendency (Rogers, 1951), 'Jennie' experienced a traumatic childhood, developing an external locus of evaluation rather than experiencing her self-worth (Rogers, 1961a). These conflicts lead to psychological difficulties of relationship losses, abandonment and distress as depicted diagrammatically later. Jennie has future plans to visit the West Indies.

**CONDITIONS OF WORTH LAID DOWN IN CHILDHOOD**
Women care for others, fear, poverty, racism
Child carer, neglect, addiction
incongruence, conditional regard, judgement

**INTROJECTED VALUES AND BELIEFS**
Most others untrustworthy, people out to hurt me
My needs come second, I blame myself
No one cares about me,
I am of less worth because I am black

**DENIAL AND DISTORTION OF EXPERIENCE**
Unworthy of love, blames herself for family unhappiness
Need for close and confiding relationships
I have to pay for love, denial of genuine true self

**STATE OF INCONGRUENCE**
Despite professional and family achievements, unlovable and unworthy
Successful career with external locus of evaluation,
Need for others to understand and care; pushes people away.

**PSYCHOLOGICAL DIFFICULTIES**
Abandonment, bewilderment, loneliness.

*Figure 6.1* Theoretical framework for embedding 'Jennie's' material into a person-centred case formulation of psychological difficulties

*Source*: Simms (2011)

The critical incidents contributing to 'Jennie's' state of incongruence are her parents' deaths, mental health, safeguarding issues and Covid-19.

## Intervention – transcript and commentary

### *Outline of the context of the recorded extract*

Jennie was admitted to a hospital with a diagnosis of bipolar type II relapse, under Section 2 of the Mental Health Act (1983). My therapeutic work with 'Jennie' comprised nine sessions; 'Jennie' was discharged after session five and readmitted a fortnight later due to noncompliance of medication (risperidone), therapy resuming with session six later. The current issues were 'Jennie's' distress on readmission, suicidal ideation and grieving.

| *Dialogue* | *Process comments*[3] |
|---|---|
| **Cl. 1** (Cries)<br>**Co. 1** I'm going to get some tissues. You make yourself comfortable (Cl. goes into quiet room; Co. goes to collect tissues from nursing station, then returns to the quiet room).<br>[Another patient asks Co. for something, and Co. responds: 'Sorry, can you just wait until the nurse comes, sorry'.]<br>Okay (I close door, 'T' is crying, mouth open, looking towards me). It's okay. I remember you [inaudible]. | I feel deeply empathic of 'Jennie's' losses (Rogers, 1957). I clear a space for 'Jennie' to share, feeling attuned to 'Jennie's' abandonment but maintaining boundaries.<br>I support 'Jennie's' focus directly on the concretely felt experience she has in the immediate moment (Rogers et al., 1967). I wonder: 'Was leaving "Jennie" an enactment, just as her parents died?' Was it a rupture (Gersch et al., 2018) or a non-verbal microaggression (Cook & O'Hara, 2020)?<br>I offer external comforters, acknowledging her implied affectivity and felt personal meaning(s) (Rogers, 1951) for self-actualisation in the community.[4]<br>I'm aware of the contact rupture, with 'Jennie' sobbing/vulnerable (Tronick & Weinberg, 1997), attempting to repair the disconnection (Safran et al., 2011).<br>I create a boundary with the door – protective. I remember 'Jennie', my communicating continuity of being and valuing, a stance of congruence, unconditional positive regard and empathy (Rogers, 1957). |
| **Cl. 2**: I can't breathe.<br>**Co. 2**: Here, I brought some tissues for you. | I feel sad, recalling George Floyd, empathic to 'Jennie', overriding my congruence. I sense 'Jennie' as a black woman poignantly, through unjust experiences; 'Jennie' perhaps felt threatened through unfavourable conditions (Rogers, 1980a; Chantler, 2005). Why didn't I explore the possible racial aspects? I was holding 'Jennie's' grief without imposing my thoughts.<br>I empathise with 'Jennie', offering her something soft to hold. |

*(Continued)*

(Continued)

| Dialogue | Process comments[3] |
| --- | --- |
| **Cl 3**: Thank you.<br>**Co 3**: It's okay, no worries. | Do my words accurately reflect her situation? I could have asked, 'You can't breathe?' |
| **Cl. 4**: If I tell my story, I'll be called a snitch.<br>**Co 4**: No, who by?<br>**Cl. 5:** My son and my partner.<br>**Co. 5:** No. | I experience surprise/fear at 'snitch' but remain in myself with 'Jennie'.<br>I convey surprise/disbelief – better perhaps: 'I hear you say you would be called a snitch, who by?'<br>Again, I am surprised by our differences. |
| **Cl. 6**: (Sobs) They care about me, but they put me in hospital because they became aggressive. They were aggressive, and my sons got beaten up. I told you he's got lots of wives, and the homeless sleep on my floor, on the carpet. I put up a sleeping bag. I feed them. I give them food. They love me (cries). They love me on the street, and I've got any money I give them.<br>**Co. 6**: Mmm. | I feel concern for 'Jennie's' living circumstances but psychologically hold her, offering a quiet, still presence, 'Jennie' perhaps emotionally weaving between themes.<br>'Jennie' appears paying for love, which saddens me, a possible link with her father's gambling, with no limits.<br>Perhaps, better: 'Your son and partner became aggressive. I wonder how that feels for you'. |
| **Cl. 7**: (Sobs) And I've hardly got no money for myself. My dad said, 'Have all the money'. And I said, 'No, I don't want it; you must share it with all of these children'.<br>**Co. 7**: Hmm. | I'm aware of 'Jennie' needing help, but struggle to think of something helpful to say, listening actively.<br>I respond non-verbally to 'Jennie's' distress, from a neutral stance, intending 'Jennie' to feel experientially and psychologically held (Elliott & Westwell, 2012) with her internal frame (Rogers, 1992). |
| **Cl. 8**: And there's five of us. We've always been poor. Now my brothers are rich, they don't want to know me. They invite me to their weddings and that's it, posh weddings with rich women they married, African women, but they've got long hair. And my son, my nephew is mixed race as well, like us, because we are mixed race. But it doesn't show. My dad is Indian and white, his mother was white, and my grandmother was white. She had long hair and blue eyes. I've got a picture of her. That's why C comes up. C is my granddaughter. She's half white.<br>**Co. 8**: Hmm. | I feel empathic (Rogers, 1957) towards 'Jennie's' distress, moving to pride about her brothers' wealth. I follow 'Jennie's' focus on the external locus of evaluation, cultural aspects (LO. 1, 2), sensing experiential reciprocity (Gendlin, 1964). Perhaps therapy is taking place in 'Jennie' (Rogers et al., 1967). |

*(Continued)*

(Continued)

| Dialogue | Process comments[3] |
|---|---|
| **Cl. 9**: And half-mixed race and she looks like a white child. She won't go dark, like her sister. Her sister is mixed race.<br>**Co. 9:** Mmm | 'Jennie' discusses race issues. There is psychological contact (Rogers, 1992) but discomfort, perhaps introjected oppression? (Alleyne, 2004). 'Jennie's' sharing feels 'person-to-person' (Rogers et al., 1967, p. 101).<br>I feel close to 'Jennie': present, caring, closely listening, communicating non-judgementally, unconditional positive regard (Rogers et al., 1967, pp. 102–103) and self-worth (Rogers, 1957). |
| **Cl. 10:** And she won't go dark. It's my child. I had a DNA test, and they said its mine.<br>**Co. 10:** Yeah. | Is 'Jennie' sharing about identity and belonging? Why don't I explore further? I feel confused by 'dark', interrupting my presence, bracketing these thoughts, returning to focus on 'Jennie's' experience (Cooper, 2000).<br>I could have asked 'Jennie' to say more (LO. 2). |
| **Cl. 11:** (Sobs) He's mine, so it proved that it was his child. There's always been sibling rivalry between him and his sister, who pretends she's on my side to get money, and they gave her money. And she went with the [inaudible] afterwards. And I said I go and save N (son) now (sobs). And I'm tearing myself apart for my three children because I love them and I love them. They're my children.<br>**Co. 11:** Yeah, you love your three children and your grandchildren.<br>**Cl. 12:** (Sobs) Yeah, and I'm not never going to see them before she's going to Scotland with her mum (daughter?). Her mum's Scottish. She's very pale. She tried with him for ten years and then she had enough and so she goes to live with her mum in Scotland.<br>**Co. 12:** Mmmm. | I feel empathic with 'Jennie's' sorrow.<br>I offer an 'empathic conjecture' (Elliot & Westwell, 2012), 'tearing myself apart' for her life – her children. |
| **Cl. 13:** And we carry on her life, but she doesn't really like Scotland because they are racist there (cries).<br>**Co. 13:** Hmm, yeah. | I feel loss, connecting from moment to moment with 'Jennie's' spoken felt sense of her daughter moving into harm.<br>I hold 'Jennie' with unconditional positive regard (Rogers et al., 1967, p. 105). |

*(Continued)*

(Continued)

| Dialogue | Process comments[3] |
|---|---|
| **Cl. 14:** And she's got a mixed-race child. | I notice race and skin colour as recurring themes. |
| **Co. 14:** I see. | I sense 'Jennie' needing a clear space, with presence. |
| **Cl. 15:** And she's been with a black person. | I connect with my felt sense of her racial suffering, holding eye contact and sitting with her feelings. |
| **Co. 15:** Hmm. | |
| **Cl. 16:** But she has to put up with him to get a flat. She's getting her flat. She says he phones me all the time and a couple of Thursdays and C (grandchild) is ill with her childhood. | I remain aware of 'Jennie's' possible introjected racial oppression. I offer consistent, reliable presence and psychological holding, promoting and validating her, allowing 'Jennie' apace (Elliot & Westwell, 2012, p. 6). |
| **Co. 16:** Hmm. | |
| **Cl. 17:** (Cries) And N (son) is meant to get better, but he is meant to teach her to read, and now she can't even read properly. And she doesn't know her times tables, and she can't read properly. All she does is makeup and dancing. | I feel connected with 'Jennie', sharing expansively, expanding experiencing further (Klein et al., 1969), perhaps 'Jennie' moving through feeling, amongst topics. I listen, clearing the space for 'Jennie' (Rogers et al., 1967). |
| **Co. 17:** Hmm. | |
| **Cl. 18:** That's what she wants to do. | I've a felt sense of 'Jennie' seeing her grandchildren. |
| **Co. 18:** Yeah, well, it sounds like you've really helped your grandchild. | I acknowledge 'Jennie's' strengths. |
| **Cl. 20:** I can't see my grandson now because of this pandemic. | I hold 'Jennie's' frustrations, responding minimally, communicating presence, active listening, contact and valuing. I would use the relational depth scale (Wiggins et al., 2012). |
| **Co. 20:** Yeah. | |
| **Cl. 21:** (Cries) But I feel not seeing them, but I haven't seen them for ages, only spoken to her on the phone. | I'm attuned to 'Jennie's' felt sense of losses, facilitating connection. I could have said, 'It sounds really difficult', for increased reflectivity. |
| **Co. 21:** That's really difficult for you that you can't see your grandchildren at the moment. | |
| **Cl. 22:** (Cries and nods) And I can't even see my children. They have to send me messages on because she has the welfare watching her. If she does, umm, anything wrong with the baby and learning from her because. | I'm uneasy about her daughter and social services (I take this to supervision). My internal response of holding 'Jennie' reflects my external response. I sense 'Jennie' feeling more positive. |
| **Co. 22:** Hmm. | |

*(Continued)*

(Continued)

| Dialogue | Process comments[3] |
|---|---|
| **Cl. 23:** I taught her how to breast-feed, how to express milk if you're going to let anyone else feed it.<br>**Co. 23:** Hmm. | I remain non-judgemental (Rogers, 1957), experiencing 'Jennie' expressing her contribution to the 'field of another' (Rogers, 1959). |
| **Cl. 24:** (Cries) I taught her how to change nappies, and my mum taught me. I went everywhere with my mum. She was my (sobs) . . . I-I-I love my m-m-m-mum.<br>**Co. 24:** You love your mum. | I feel moved by 'Jennie' touching losses regarding her mother.<br>My response is guided by the feelings, words, images and intuitions emerging in me from my experience of being with 'Jennie' (Geller et al., 2010; Geller, 2013), held with positive regard (Rogers et al., 1967, p. 104). |
| **Cl. 25:** (Sobs) And it's five years now, and I still go to the cemetery, they both and my dad. My dad died last year. Just before the Covid-19, he died. And my uncle died the year before. The both of them were buried together because they were Catholic.<br>**Co. 25:** Ahh. | I remain consistently still and quiet, being with her plural, relational self-entities (Cooper, 2000, p. 4).<br>My intention is to be with 'Jennie', recounting her losses perhaps for the first time, promoting her actualising tendency (Rogers, 1979, p. 2). |
| **Cl. 26:** They are Catholic, and they were both close.<br>**Co. 26:** Yeah, and so you've had 'T'. You have had quite a few losses in the last couple of years, and you said you lost, and I remember that you told me that you'd lost your father. | I acknowledge 'Jennie's' loss to process her experiences, alongside goals (Cooper & Law, 2018). I offer a focusing response, moving into hinted-at feelings for support, containing overwhelming feelings, within a safe, psychologically holding environment (Elliot & Westwell, 2012). |
| **Cl. 27:** Yeah (nods), and I loved him as well.<br>**Co. 27:** And that was just a year ago. | I encounter our poignant dialogue (Schmid, 2009), 'Jennie' communicating her father's death as a past event, adjusting her reality, through profound contact (Mearns & Cooper, 2005).<br>I support 'Jennie's' mourning. I think this evokes increased understanding and movement to something new regarding 'Jennie's' self-exploration of being and actualisation. |
| **Cl. 28:** (Cries) Yeah, it just hit me now that we won't see him anymore. We used to go every weekend to his house and cook him dinner, dance with him, make him feel young.<br>**Co. 28:** Right. | I feel the embodied impact of 'hit me now' as an empathic communication of 'Jennie's' realisations (Rogers, 1961a), connecting with her father.<br>I affirm 'Jennie' through her grieving, remaining being with her experience. What is 'Jennie' not feeling or talking about in these moments? I could have followed this experientially with emotion-focused work (Gendlin, 1981). |

*(Continued)*

(Continued)

| Dialogue | Process comments[3] |
|---|---|
| **Cl. 29:** But we knew he had cancer, and I went with him to an appointment with the consultant at [hospital]. And then one day, he phoned me up, and I went round. And there's vomiting all black stuff. And I phoned an ambulance, and they came and took him into hospital and said that he is getting worse.<br>**Co. 29:** Right. | I notice 'Jennie's' repetition of 'we' – her social self. I wonder what the ongoing feeling process is now. How can it be facilitated therapeutically (Rogers et al., 1967)?<br>I feel prizing of 'Jennie' and stay with this experience of profound contact (Mearns & Cooper, 2018). |
| **Cl. 30:** And they kept him there and that's when I ended up in here, and I said, 'Well, it's only across the road. I can see him.' And they said I couldn't because it's only going to upset you more (pause).<br>**Co. 30:** I see. | I'm aware of my internal flow of experiencing, 'Jennie' becoming unwell prior to her father's death for connection – perhaps for repair, or to join him in death?<br>I sense my response as congruent regarding what I was taking in from being with 'Jennie'. |
| **Cl. 31:** And took him to [another hospital]. I said, 'Why? Why?'<br>**Co. 31:** Are you saying that the medical staff, um. | The interaction between 'Jennie' and I felt flowing and rhythmic, empathically aware of 'Jennie's' vulnerability, like a child demanding, 'Why is this happening?' |
| **Cl. 32:** They wouldn't let me go across the road to visit my dad.<br>**Co. 32:** They didn't want you to see him because they thought it would upset you.<br>**Cl. 33:** Because I was crying here.<br>**Co: 33:** Right. | I felt conflicted in the moment.<br>I offer a different perspective, but this moves away from meeting 'Jennie' in an immediate, personal encounter, verbalising her present, personal meaning, with 'Jennie's' feeling as central. I could have said, 'I wonder how you felt about that'.<br>I feel surprise again by the past meeting the present.<br>I'm sensing 'Jennie' being brought to the edge of awareness. |
| **Cl. 34:** (Cries) I thought I would go and see my dad; it was my idea to write a will. But I thought he was going to write it for just for everyone. But he was leaving my brother out. But I said, 'No, don't leave it for all of us'.<br>**Co. 34:** Are you saying that you didn't have your chance to say goodbye? | I feel prizing of 'Jennie' (Rogers, 1957), sticking by her brother. I move into hinted-at feelings, regarding not saying goodbye, trying to verbalise 'Jennie's' implicit meanings.<br>I track 'Jennie's' internal frame of reference and response, creating a profound moment of deep understanding (RDFS-C, point 3, Wiggins et al., 2012). |
| **Cl. 35:** Yeah.<br>**Co. 35:** I see, okay. | I felt alert and attuned to the nuances of 'Jennie's' experiences, affirming a sense of understanding her struggle with existential issues (Spinelli, 2014). We work as Thou-I (Schmid, 2006) alongside 'ethics in action' (Cooper, 2009, p. 120), towards actualisation (Rogers, 1959, 1980a). |

*(Continued)*

(Continued)

| Dialogue | Process comments[3] |
|---|---|
| **Cl. 36:** I was starting to, me and V (sister) did the burial and everything and organising it.<br>**Co. 36:** Mmm, and what would you want to say? What would you have wanted to say to your father to say goodbye? | I feel deeply engaged and in contact with 'Jennie'.<br>I connect with an implied sense of 'Jennie' wanting to say goodbye to her father, for closure, offering experiential specificity (Elliot & Creswell, 2012). |
| **Cl. 37:** Just thank you.<br>**Co. 37:** Thank you. | I felt attuned to 'Jennie'.<br>I reflect 'Jennie's' words to enhance my relational presence (Rogers, 1973) in this poignant moment. I empathise, reflecting 'Jennie's' feelings (Rogers, 2002, p. 13) as a response process (Temaner, 1977). |
| **Cl. 38:** Thank you for [inaudible tears] because it was worse in the '60s and '70s than it is now because there was more racism. And my mum and dad used to try to like people and me. And I was just a little girl. And they wanted me to [inaudible tears] because I was, I had long hair down to my waist, and I cut it all once to give to my mum to wear as a wig. And she didn't like me doing that.<br>**Co. 38:** I see, so you cut your own hair so that your mother could have a wig. | I experience an ongoing feeling process of deep sorrow in these moments of movement – 'Jennie' recalling experiencing her parents trying to like people in the face of racism. I think of 'Jennie's' direct feeling now, reminding of a 'direct referent' and the emotional movement (Gendlin & Zimberg, 1955; Rogers, 1958, 1960). I held 'Jennie's' sorrow and returning to a challenging ward.<br>I feel moved and imagine 'Jennie' feeling the same way (point four on the relational depth frequency scale? Wiggins et al., 2012). I stay with 'Jennie's' frame of reference. |
| **Cl. 39:** All her hair's falling out, and all my hair's falling out, so I'm stressed.<br>**Co. 39:** Your hair, it's really nice. | I notice 'Jennie' referring to her mother in the present, coming alive in her mind. I would have explored 'Jennie's' feeling of stress in an embodied way, 'I wonder where you feel your stress' (Gendlin, 1981). I hear the nurse approaching and follow 'Jennie'. I could have been congruent, saying, 'I hear the nurse approaching'. |
| **Cl. 40:** Yeah, curly.<br>**Co. 40:** Really curly. | I feel conflicted, anticipating this situation.<br>I psychologically hold 'Jennie' positively but feel incongruent. |
| **Cl. 41:** Naturally curly, but I can have it straight if I blow-dry it. The hairdresser came and did it.<br>**Co. 41:** Oh, really? | I reflect on 'Jennie's' hair perhaps symbolising her identity and culture, with choices. |
| **Cl. 42:** It looked so good, shiny.<br>**Co. 42:** Yeah. | I notice 'Jennie's' pride in her shiny hair. My response is minimal, psychologically holding the space for 'Jennie'. |

*(Continued)*

(Continued)

| Dialogue | Process comments[3] |
|---|---|
| **Cl. 43:** And no need to straighten it. It's a blow-dry.<br>**Co. 43:** So you can choose whether you have straight hair or curly hair. | I consider that I convey unconditional acceptance, being centred in myself, alongside my felt sense of 'Jennie's' intense vulnerability (Elliott & Westwell, 2012).<br>I'm prizing of 'Jennie's' culture – her perceived belonging with black-and-white cultures? |
| **Cl. 44:** I can go out with it wet, and it goes curly.<br>**Co. 44:** Okay. | I continue to track 'Jennie's' frame of reference and self-concept, accepting 'Jennie' and trying to facilitate the core conditions (Rogers, 1957, 1980b). I consistently follow 'Jennie's' lead when responding to content in a natural, inviting and unforced manner (Elliot & Westwell, 2012, pp. 2–3). |
| **Cl. 45:** I can spray water on it. I don't even need to use products. All these expensive products that people use to make their hair go curly, I don't need to. I just wash it and dry it, and it goes curly.<br>**Co. 45:** Yeah, you're lucky. | I consistently promote and affirm 'Jennie's' autonomy, allowing 'Jennie' space as she desires (Elliot & Westwell, 2012, p. 3). I follow 'Jennie's' felt meaning, alongside verbal content. I notice her mood shift from sorrow to empowerment. |
| **Cl. 46:** I know that's what everyone says. It's because of my dad.<br>**Co. 46:** Sure. | I notice 'Jennie' expressing an external locus of evaluation. I wonder if 'Jennie' wanting to straighten her hair is related to internalised oppression (Alleyne, 2004).<br>Incongruently, I experience anxiety as the nurse approaches and express certainty to 'Jennie', appearing unaware of the nurse outside. |
| [Knock on door. Nurse opens door with her keys and enters.]<br>**Nurse:** Sorry to interrupt, just to give 'T' her medication.<br>**Co. 47:** Sure. | I feel present but annoyed at the nurse's intrusion, my mind focusing on 'Jennie's' needs.<br>I offer certainty to help provide her with psychological holding. |
| **Cl. 48:** This medication is not doing anything for me. It's just making me cry all the time.<br>**Nurse:** It's not the medication that's making you cry, 'T'.<br>**Cl. 49:** It's my condition then. They say I'm bipolar.<br>(Pause)<br>**Co. 49:** Maybe it's. | I remain quiet, as an observer-participant, supporting the medication exchange, involving control and power. I notice 'Jennie's' aggression here.<br>I notice 'Jennie' backtrack on her aggression.<br>I feel conflicted, attempting mediation; the nurse asserts containment. |
| **Nurse:** (to Cl.) Do you want some water?<br>**Cl. 50:** I've got a broken heart.<br>**Co. 50:** Maybe it's your broken heart, but we're talking about that, aren't we, you and I? | I feel attuned to 'Jennie's' 'broken heart', offering psychological holding. |

*(Continued)*

(Continued)

| Dialogue | Process comments[3] |
|---|---|
| **Cl. 51:** There's such a thing that you can die from (sobs).<br>**Co. 51:** Thank you [to nurse who leaves and closes the door]. | I was aware of my own internal flow of experiencing sorrow at 'Jennie's' expression of brokenness and invalidation. I feel this rupture. 'Jennie's' mood moves from pride to disbelief. |
| **Cl. 52:** (Cries) People don't think that it's true.<br>**Co. 52:** It's really difficult, 'T', when your father only died a year ago. | I feel saddened by 'Jennie's' despair.<br>I focus on 'Jennie's' core meaning and pain, a response guided by her feelings and words, alongside my intuitions, sharing with 'Jennie'. |
| **Co. 53:** And then they left all the pictures of him with me and 'N' and 'J' and 'J' my children and keeping him happy, going swimming with him and anything that he would like, playing jazz at home and dancing to it. They used to show him how they danced because they are dancers. I wanted them to be famous, like The Jackson 5 (cries), but they never learned to sing. | The dialogue between 'Jennie' and I feel emotionally flowing, deep and rhythmic. |

## Endings

I attempted emotionally staying with Jennie's distress every step of the way, from moment-to-moment presence; Jennie's sobbing subsided towards the end of this session. Jennie was prompted ten minutes prior to ending, supporting her to return to the ward. As Jennie was accompanied back, she mentioned feeling better having cried and talked things through. 'Jennie' noticeably appeared more grounded with her complexion glowing.

## Evaluation

This sixth session appeared to facilitate Jennie's felt experiencing of distress regarding her section under the Mental Health Act (1983); the main goal of the therapy, as articulated by Jennie, was to talk through her grieving. An aim was to psychologically hold (Elliott & Westwell, 2012) Jennie with my benign presence, within the seven stages of process change (Rogers, 1961a), six necessary and sufficient conditions (Rogers, 1992), alongside Rogers's nineteen propositions of personality change (Rogers, 1992). No one wanted to listen to Jennie, but a space was cleared to support her letting me know her towards an experiential focus (Gendlin, 1981). I struggled regarding how to best work with Jennie's vulnerability, from a person-centred perspective, wondering whether Jennie's 'bipolar' condition is secondary to her abuses. Jennie's 'bipolar' condition appeared psychogenic; the abuses, alcoholic father, etc., perhaps disturbed her chemically. It was clear that Jennie was very distressed in her mid-sixties, grieving her losses prompted by the death of her parents. This work was supported by group supervision, the ward staff, one-to-one supervision and personal therapy.

Perhaps complex Post Traumatic Stress Disorder in ICD-11 (World Health Organisation, 2019) would be a more appropriate understanding of Jennie's situation in medical and psychological terms. In formulating Jennie's situation, alternately, her mother's protection has ceased since she died; Jennie's support system has fallen away. Jennie conveys her 'broken heart', witnessing her father destroying himself through drinking and having another partner abroad. 'Jennie' experienced a lot of abuse secondary to what she was exposed to with her father, alongside possible genderised and racialised conditions of worth (Chantler, 2005). Her husband and partner reportedly raped her. Her son is abusive, inviting her ex-partner into her home. Her parents died, leading to a breakdown, her distress symbolising much conflict in her life (Cromby et al., 2013).

Jennie's literal felt meanings were responded to, including her pre-verbal, pre-conceptual experiencing, encouraging Jennie to focus directly on the concretely felt experience in the immediate moment, for verbalisation (Rogers et al., 1967, p. 370). Evoked feelings were reflected upon, via Jennie's raw feelings of loss, maintaining my presence through intense sessions, amidst challenging ward interruptions. My Covid-19 mask covered half of my face, which was discussed with her.

Mostly, Jennie was offered congruence, unconditional positive regard and empathy. These conditions provided an actualising direction (Cooper, 2021) for Jennie, feeling safe to grieve, despite intrusions, raising ethical issues of confidentiality and safety, whilst modulating Jennie's intensity of distress (Warner, 2013, p. 348). It was difficult offering a person-centred therapy on a psychosis unit regarding case management aspects, including the demands of the ward and client, at times overriding therapeutic focus. These aspects sometimes influenced the therapeutic relationship more than perhaps realised at the time, regarding managing the spheres of medical model and therapy.

Focusing on Jennie's grieving was perhaps prioritised over, for instance, reflecting her feelings (Rogers, 1942) regarding race, in my counsellor responses 2, 8, 9, 10, 13, 14 and 38. This possibly created limitations, possibly restricting Jennie's emotional expression about race and being understood, alongside my not practising hospitalisation (Spinelli, 2005). The important cultural theme of 'Jennie's' hair was acknowledged, but the meaning for her could have been explored more. I recognised Jennie's need for closure with her father, offering her appropriate opportunity to experience saying goodbye.

The formulation process (Simms, 2011) was helpful for considering 'Jennie's' developmental emotional needs across her lifespan. The Simms's model (2011) leaves out protective factors and power/threat issues (Johnstone & Boyle, 2018), with elements overlapping in different sense.

I explored, under supervision, whether it is person-centred to take up the moment of 'Jennie's' aggression when the nurse entered, as well as regarding 'Jennie's' daughter and baby. Personal therapy facilitated reflexivity regarding my incongruence during this session. In this clip, Jennie' poured out her 'broken heart'; on the ward, people felt flooded and moved away or diagnosed her. I focused on what is central to 'Jennie'. Jennie appeared to need attention regarding her life losses and achievements, and she was vulnerable. Jennie seemed to create particular relationships, where she overwhelmed others and, at times, ignored my mind. There was no shortage of experiences evoking in Jennie's mind: race, children, broken heart, pictures of her father, but at times, it was hard to get in and say anything to her.

Following session nine, Jennie withdrew from therapy, and a change of medication coincided with her being less disinhibited: How could empathy provide an internal locus of self-worth in person-centred therapy in contrast to what she has introjected? My reflections hoped to progress the meaning of whatever is gained from the empathy and to build her story with me in therapy for personality change (Rogers, 1958, p. 142) in relation to the 'Process Scale' (Rogers & Rablen, 1958). There appeared contradictions regarding 'Jennie' talking about racial harmony and her problematic family. Jennie experienced 'a very difficult life' but hoped to return to the West Indies to have a happy ending. 'Jennie' is on my mind often, hoping that she is well.

## Notes

1 This concept would readily translate to the psychoanalytic thinking of 'sense of self', in my opinion. This point highlights the many overlaps between so-called differently named therapeutic approaches and undermines the territoriality often emerging between so-named different modalities. Jennie spoke about 'one love', with relevance for psychotherapy.

2 A nurse reported Jennie being violent towards her. Subsequently, I sat near the door in the consulting room, equipped with an Absco alarm. Two metres of social distance were required due to Covid-19 guidelines.

3 'Jennie' is a pseudonym used to protect the confidentiality and privacy of the client.

4 I envisage self-actualisation as the ongoing lifelong process whereby an individual's self-concept is sustained and enhanced through reflection, alongside the reinterpretation of various experiences, enabling the individual to recover, change and develop (Rogers, 1951), tentatively holding the self-concept (Rogers, 1961a, 1961b).

# 7 Assessment case study 3 – 'Sandra'

To-morrow, and to-morrow, and to-morrow,
Creeps in this petty pace from day to day,
To the last syllable of recorded time;
And all our yesterdays have lighted fools
The way to dusty death. Out, out, brief candle!
Life's but a walking shadow, a poor player,
That struts and frets his hour upon the stage,
And then is heard no more.

*Macbeth*, Act V, Scene V, Line 19–28

## Assessment

### Context and referral

'Sandra' sought therapy when she self-referred to a female acute ward, presenting in crisis as self-neglecting alongside low mood, anxiety, alcohol misuse, self-harm and suicidal ideation. She was then referred to me for assessment. Previously, Sandra received weekly sessions with a psychotherapist referred through a different service, which she found helpful but was unfinished due to the therapist leaving. I discovered that Sandra had, in fact, been refused continuation of therapy, seemingly due to her arriving late to two of the therapy sessions offered. This situation appeared perplexing to me, and I wondered why the situation had not been managed differently within the team. Upon further exploration, there appeared to have been an unhelpful enactment, where Sandra was uncontained and the psychotherapist responded dismissively, perhaps with a lack of supervision and a team to support their work with Sandra.

### Introducing Sandra

In therapy, it is a core skill to facilitate accurate collaborative assessments and formulations, with awareness of limitations (Groth-Marnat, 2003, p. 1),

DOI: 10.4324/9781003509059-8

including Covid-19 guidance (British Psychological Society (BPS), 2020, 2021). A phenomenological stance embodies the humanistic and relational philosophy and values of therapy, describing clients' experiences in their own words (Husserl, 1969). Self-reflexivity is central when assessing individuals, tracing subjectivity, intersubjectivity, spatiality, embodiment and imagination (Zahavi, 2018, p. 2). The individual seeks help as an active agent (Bohart & Tallman, 1999), co-creating meaning within social-cultural-political contexts (Horvath & Greenberg, 1994). An assessment intends to explore the client's psychological contact, goals for therapy, risk/safeguarding, interventions, lifespan stage and preferences (Carter & McGoldrick, 2004) for agency, security, connection, meaning, trust – actualisation (Rogers, 1951, p. 487). The person-centred approach upholds three main strands, namely, Rogers' nineteen propositions (1951), seven stages of process (1961a) and six necessary and sufficient conditions for therapeutic personality change (1992), interwoven into this assessment process alongside the Simms (2011) formulation model.

Conducting an effective, ethical, psychological assessment from a stance embodying the philosophy and values of therapy may involve six values (Orlans & Van Scoyoc, 2008; Woolfe, 1996): initially, highlighting the client's subjective and intersubjective experiences, compared to the therapist's observations or outcome measures; secondly, prioritising facilitating growth and development alongside actualising potential, in contrast to psychopathology; thirdly, empowering clients; fourthly, an adherence to a fair, equitable, client-therapist relationship, with the client as expert; fifthly, acknowledging the client's uniqueness, compared to an example of universal laws; and sixthly, comprehending the client as a socially and relationally orientated individual, alongside awareness regarding the client possibly experiencing prejudices and discrimination versus an entirely internal focus (Orlans & Van Scoyoc, 2008; Woolfe, 1996).

In attempting to bring the assessment closer to the client's subjectivity, intersubjectivity, values and feelings, the client is positioned as expert for ethical mutuality, enhancing autonomy and their internal frame of reference (Rogers, 1951, p. 29). Covid-19 restrictions prescribed online assessments, facilitated according to British Psychological Society guidance (2020, 2021) with various challenges. Selected cultural and sociopolitical psychological assessment methods informed the process with 'Sandra'. For example, Engel's biopsychosocial model (Engel, 1977; Adler, 2009) relates to the NHS and the power-threat-meaning-framework (PTMF) (Johnstone & Boyle, 2018), illuminated aspects of power alongside forms of and responses to threat. Bronfenbrenner's (1977) ecological model contextualised 'Sandra' in society; social justice models such as Kagan et al. (2011), Goodman et al. (2004) and McClelland (2014) contributed respectively, for instance, peacefulness, strengths and consciousness. Additionally, neuroscience assists the understanding of brain science and depression, for example, alongside neuropsychological assessments, such as Wechsler Memory Scales (Wechsler, 1997). Neuroscience and scales surely distract from focusing on the client's perspective to within their own terms of reference. However, recent research helpfully integrates neuroscience into counselling psychology (Goss, 2016).

The assessment and formulation of 'Sandra' involved managing various conflicting information, guidance and regulation regarding the relevance of diagnosis, considered ethically in relation to the client's best interests. According to Bor and Watts (2017), the process of assessment involves 'negotiating the movement between the client's frames of reference, the therapist's frames of reference and the context in a way that does not violate this ethic' (Bor & Watts, 2017, p. 295), which appears appropriate. Let us now turn to the assessment of 'Sandra'.

### Referral and context

'Sandra' sought therapy on the acute ward and was referred to me for assessment. The consultant ward psychiatrist assessed that 'Sandra' had the mental capacity to consent to sharing her personal data. A collaborative assessment of 'Sandra's' capacity to consent was facilitated by me to use written material from her assessments for publication, including transcribed extracts. The General Data Protection Regulation (Data Protection Act, 2020) guidance on confidentiality and storage was detailed to 'Sandra'. 'Sandra' and I assessed that she had the mental capacity (Mental Capacity Act, 2005) to understand, retain, weigh up and communicate this information, and she consented. I handed the consent form to her, and 'Sandra' returned the signed consent form, then being stored in a locked cabinet.

The client perspective outcome measure webforms were handed to 'Sandra', namely, PHQ-9 (Kroenke et al., 2001), GAD-7 (Spitzer et al., 2006) and WSAS (Mundt et al., 2002).[1] Forms were completed and returned by 'Sandra' prior to the first assessment and before and after the second assessment. 'Sandra's' reason for seeking support was an initial diagnosis of 'major recurrent depressive disorder' ICD-10 F33 (World Health Organisation (WHO), 1993). Her experiences involved the following: 'low mood, anxiety and self-harm including overdoses and suicidal ideation since adolescence . . . triggered by negative early experiences'. Following 'Sandra's' assessments with me, a different diagnosis of 'childhood emotional disorder' ICD-10 F93.9 (WHO, 1993) was given from a senior psychotherapist.

Initially, the boundaries of the assessment relationship were clarified, whilst curious to engage with 'Sandra' in dialogue. 'Sandra' described feeling 'unhappy most of the time', regarding her 'appearance and not being good enough and failing'. A recent onset involved her healthcare training, finding it 'difficult to complete assignments' due to 'mood swings and negative thoughts, lack of concentration, loss of appetite, using alcohol to relax', increasing difficulties 'with anxiety, sleeping and low mood'. 'Sandra' described her previous experience of psychotherapy, which was unfinished due to the therapist leaving. 'Sandra' relayed a history of unsustained psychotherapy but feeling ready to commit now.

### Background and presentation

'Sandra' is a well-presented early 30-year-old mixed-race woman struggling to complete her healthcare training. Her mother is 'white-British', her father 'black-Indian'. 'Sandra' described her father as alcoholic, recalling from childhood being frightened because he was emotionally and physically abusive, calling her 'slut' and 'prostitute'. Her parents divorced at her age of 14, sharing the same house until 'Sandra' was 17 years old. Then her mother started drinking heavily. 'Sandra' started seeking out dangerous company, being raped repeatedly and her life threatened. 'Sandra' described returning home with ripped clothes and bruises, but her mother ignored this, which she remains angry about. However, 'Sandra' communicated having a 'good' relationship generally with her mother, 'despite not being able to rely on her' to meet her emotional needs. 'Sandra' portrayed an improved relationship with her father, but he continues making 'hurtful comments', such as encouraging her to end her life.

'Sandra' was punctual for both assessments, with clean-appearing and casual presentation, sounding slurred in speech, at times nervous but sharing openly with me.

'Sandra's' outcome measure scores:

Preceding first assessment: PHQ-9 = 24/27 severe depression, GAD-7 = 20/21 severe anxiety and WSAS = 32 severe interference with daily tasks.

Preceding second assessment: PHQ-9 = 22/27 severe depression and GAD-7 = 18/21 severe anxiety.

One week proceeding second assessment: PHQ-9 = 19/27 severe depression and GAD-7 = 16/21 severe anxiety.

'Sandra' considered these scores highlighting her 'isolation and difficulty with coping', alongside 'I feel listened to' improving her scores. When discussing her suicidal ideation, 'Sandra' became very tearful, considering her mother the only person who would care if she died.

### Current situation

'Sandra' is single and currently unemployed, although she has offers of employment as a healthcare worker once qualified. She conveyed separating from a married man a month ago, telling him to contact her once he has left his marriage; when 'Sandra's' mood became 'very low', she heard voices telling her to take her own life, and she lost her 'motivation' taking 'an intentional overdose' of various pills to 'stop the emotional pain rather than to die'. 'Sandra' considered this relationship unhealthy but would take him back if the opportunity arose. 'Sandra' described becoming increasingly isolated with friends but finding it difficult because of her depressed mood. 'Sandra' had lived unhappily in a hospital accommodation as a healthcare worker, with tradesmen currently entering her halls of residence to make repairs at any time. Sandra's voices had grown more intrusive, and she volunteered herself into an inpatient ward.

### The meeting

'Sandra' appeared very low in mood, especially at the first assessment, when describing her recent relationship break-up and hearing voices to take her own life. 'Sandra' reported having a positive relationship with her two sisters, though stating that they are both 'very introverted', and her mother who helps her.

In the second assessment, 'Sandra' described going into the world when she was 13, whilst her mother and father fought and her mother was drinking heavily, finding men who sexually exploited her. Once, two men approached her in the park at night and held a screwdriver to her, stating they would kill her; one sexually assaulted her, the other refusing to do so. On other occasions, 'Sandra' described a man punching her repeatedly in the face in the street, dragging her to a grass area and repeatedly sexually assaulting her. She returned to this group of men, who exploited her and threatened her life, putting her in a van boot and covering her in petrol.

'Sandra' appeared very tearful at the thought of her dying. The degree of 'Sandra's' emotional neglect was clear. 'Sandra' described lacking guidance and protection through adolescence, going out into the world, seeking care and attention but meeting with horrific experiences and having no one to talk to about it or to seek comfort from. Aware of feeling protective towards 'Sandra', I experienced haunting images of her at risk.

### Strengths and resources

'Sandra' referred to her mother and sisters as support, with limitations, her sisters being 'introverted' and her mother 'heavily drinking'. There is a lack of a support network due to 'Sandra's' low mood.

### Client's aims

'Sandra' explored her preferences for change in psychotherapy described as 1) to feel happier and improve her low mood, 2) to improve her self-esteem, 3) to feel better about her body image since her eating habits fluctuate and 4) to feel more emotionally stable and to explore her past and current difficulties with relationships, especially with men.

**Formulation**

This collaborative formulation (British Psychological Society, 2011, 2017) with 'Sandra' summarises a shared understanding of her difficulties within the person-centred model (Simms, 2011). Due to the 'non-directive' philosophy underpinning the person-centred approach, Rogers (1951) rejected case formulation, believing it created power inequalities in the therapeutic relationship towards the therapist as expert, with the potential to cause harm (Eels, 2007; Johnstone & Dallos, 2014, p. 216). Gillon (2012) critiqued Simms's (2011) model regarding its linearity and lack of collaboration. HCPC (2015) considers formulation assisting multi-disciplinary work, communication supporting and revising client lived experiences and assessing and planning interventions as scientist-reflective practitioners (Challoner & Papayianni, 2012, p. 48).

During the first and especially second assessment, 'Sandra' and I had bonded, discussing her needs warmly and openly, with 'Sandra' conveying feeling safe with me. In person-centred terms, it appears that Sandra's conditions of worth (Rogers, 1951) laid down in childhood were that females are worthless and sexual objects, love is abusive, and 'Sandra' is not worth attending to. The concomitant introjected values and beliefs are that 'Sandra' is worthless, abuse equals love, and she doesn't deserve life. 'Sandra's' actualising tendency (Rogers, 1957) had been thwarted through her father's abusive comments, alongside a lack of love, appropriate attention and parental protection, comprising neglect.

In terms of denial and distortion 'Sandra' denied her needs, considering abuse the same as love and care, seeking this in the world, leading to further hurt, using alcohol and overdoses to cope rather than intending to die. 'Sandra' communicated difficulty in facing her mother's neglect of her needs. Subsequently, 'Sandra' is in a state of incongruence, feeling anxious, low, vulnerable, exploited and in danger. This leaves 'Sandra' with severe psychological difficulties, such as hurt, distress, severe anxiety, low mood and her competencies and career compromised. 'Sandra' continues having unhealthy relationships with men. She feels unsafe in her home, linked to her profession, where workmen enter and exit without her permission, indicating her emotional vulnerability and social withdrawal as coping mechanisms. This perhaps symbolises her past – that people can do what they want to her. In order to self-soothe, 'Sandra' drinks alcohol, leading to the numbing of her affect. 'Sandra' brought other people's views of herself, struggling to convey what she thought and felt, expressing an external locus of evaluation. Additionally, 'Sandra' appears distracted and traumatised, vulnerable to exploitation. This perhaps links with unspoken feelings of depression, anxiety, anger, guilt and powerlessness. It appears important for 'Sandra' to discuss her loss of partner and her past, indicative of a sense of self that needs to strengthen, grow and develop. 'Sandra' spoke of self-harming in the past by cutting but continues to use alcohol, as depicted in the following figure.

**Conditions of worth laid down in childhood**
Females are worthless, females are sexual objects, abuse equals love.

**Introjected values and beliefs**
Being female is worthless, females gain love through abuse, females aren't worth attending to,
'Sandra' deserves to be abused; life isn't worth living.

**Denial and distortion of experience**
Mistrust of the organismic valuing system, thwarting of the actualising tendency, engaging in abusive relationships to prove self worthless, alcohol numbs feelings.

**State of incongruence**
Denial of emotional needs leading to psychological difficulties.

**Psychological difficulties**
Low mood, despair, suicidal ideation, fear, anger.

*Figure 7.1* Theoretical framework for embedding client material into a person-centred case formulation of psychological difficulties

The critical incidents include the developmental stages of childhood and adolescence, involving verbal and physical abuse from her father, alcoholism and parental divorce, as well as young adulthood, involving seeking out abusive situations endangering her life, currently living alone in unsafe circumstances, using alcohol, interrupted career and terminated partnership. The self 'Sandra' presents to the world is vulnerable, isolated and at risk of suicide.

### Evaluation

The assessment and formulation experience are often recollected by clients as significant regarding their therapeutic journey, both as an event and a process, facilitated sometimes by a separate practitioner. Therefore, limitations to the assessment relationship need clarifying to contain emotional confusion. Having positively co-assessed 'Sandra's' capacity to consent, it was also communicated that General Data Protection Regulations (DPA, 2020, GDPR, 2025). Please correct the callout or add the missing Reference. state that data can be stored for no longer than necessary for the task performed.

During the assessment process with 'Sandra', Rogers's (1961a) seven stages of process of change, six necessary and sufficient conditions (Rogers, 1957) and nineteen propositions of personality change (Rogers, 1992) facilitated the assessment of 'Sandra's' potential for relationship. The conditions of worth were facilitative (Rogers, 1951) – 'Sandra' feeling safe enough to share with me, particularly in the second meeting. I gently conveyed to 'Sandra' that she would be referred to a psychologist by me. My active and authentic encounter with 'Sandra' in the here and now reminded me of Buber's (1970) description of the I-Thou relationship. Psychological contact was readily established and maintained with 'Sandra' (Rogers, 1956), although, sometimes, she appeared emotionally disconnected, vague and overwhelmed. 'Sandra' appeared able to receive the core conditions (Rogers, 1957), although perhaps struggling to negotiate the emotional proximity between us, which the organismic valuing process perhaps evoked in her (Rogers, 1959). I invited Sandra to the ward therapy group that I facilitated and she attended, appearing quietly disoriented and extremely vulnerable to people saying and doing what they wanted to her.

Working on wards demands additional governance of attempted 'objectivity'. Psychometric tests arguably offer opportunities for the client's perspective to be shared, with the assessor's presence and authentic curiosity, opening a transparent dialogue. Clinical outcome measures, such as PHQ-9 (Kroenke et al., 2001), fulfil funding requirements for evidence-based practice, alongside providing a convenient means for conceptualising effectiveness, as highlighted by the National Institute of Clinical Excellence (NICE, 2007). PHQ-9 and GAD-7 standardised measurements are usually now applied fortnightly. CORE-10 (Barkham et al., 2013) would have better replaced the outcome measure offered to 'Sandra' to not overwhelm her. To what extent, however, is the NICE research in touch with practice? The person-centred practitioner inevitably becomes drawn towards diagnosis and client improvement regarding symptom reduction (Bor & Watts, 2017). Although outcome measures may offer a convenient 'objective' evidence-base for distress, they may distract

clients from naturally expressing themselves and from the therapeutic relationship. The WSAS outcome measure during Covid-19, facilitated discussion
of 'Sandra's' situation but may have been inappropriate. Rogers insightfully
stated, 'in a very meaningful way therapy is diagnosis' (Rogers, 1951, p. 22).

Alternately, these idiographic outcome measures, emphasising the meas-
urement and analysis of variables for 'Sandra', compared to nomothetic
research strategies focusing on identifying covariations between variables
using data from groups, appeared helpful for assessing risk with her. Bozarth
(1998 advocated for psychometric assessments within 'the framework of the
therapist's dedication to the client's world and self-authority' (p. 128) with
increased reliability and validity. It appears helpful to discuss more fully the
client's experiences of such measures.

Studies by Bieling and Kukyen (2003) and Eels and Lombart (2003) compared formulation accuracy and validity, whilst Flinn et al. (2015) examined
formulation reliability, Mumma (2011) discussed issues of limitations and
validity. 'Sandra' consistently expressed experiencing suicidal thoughts and
feelings, with a thought-plan for suicide by hanging or overdose but denying
any intentional plan – her protective factor being her mother. 'Sandra' and
I assessed moderate risk of harm to self and from others, yet my supervisor
considered her at low risk, with no suicide plan.

'Sandra' demonstrated possible signs of alcoholism, drinking every day,
alongside considerations of increased risk regarding substance misuse with
possible medication and past overdosing. 'Sandra's' perception may be
different to mine, for example, regarding suicidality, which was discussed
in supervision. The relational components of person-centred assessment
and formulation processes inform a corroborative and responsive
phenomenological approach to the client's developing processes of change
(Tufekcioglu & Muran, 2015). A care plan was agreed upon, including
accessing Accident and Emergency, the Samaritans and the telephone
numbers were sent to 'Sandra'.

'Sandra's' outcome scores improved, unsurprising perhaps since she
responded well to appropriate attention yet was untrusting of non-professionals
from whom she could gain additional support. It was 'Sandra's' improved
mood that indicated progress, alongside the scores. It is in all our interests to
improve the client experience through the assessment and formulation process, perhaps by advocating the use of and developing a wider range of experiential measures (Freire et al., 2007; Wiggins et al., 2012), alongside guidance
to develop the evidence-base further in the person-centred community.

Defining clients' experiences through DSM-V T-R (American Psychiatric
Association (APA), 2013) or ICD-10 (World Health Organisation (WHO),
1993) and creating a treatment plan denies the evolving nature of the actualising tendency towards an internal locus of evaluation (Mearns & Thorne, 2000).
'Sandra's' strengths and resources were discussed, rather than focusing on deficits, inspired by Rogers's replacing diagnosis with empathic understanding.

'Sandra' arrived with a diagnosis of 'schizoaffective disorder', perhaps having an impact in itself – the issue of the referring person's opinion influencing the client's life course (Palazolli et al., 1980). When discussing 'Sandra's' recent diagnosis from a senior psychotherapist, using ICD-10, F93.9 of 'childhood emotional disorder', 'Sandra' perhaps unquestioningly accepted this. Both diagnoses convey little about the aetiology and are confusing. Social constructionism invites questions, such as this: How can we bring the client into the process (Gergen et al., 1996)? However, individuals need a diagnosis for various reasons: insurance, benefit income, acknowledgement, etc.

Regarding psychopharmacology, it is unclear what medication, if any, 'Sandra' had been prescribed and who assessed her initially. It appears that anti-psychotic and anti-depressant medication may have a certain effect to help 'Sandra', but her level of alcohol intake is an increased risk. In light of her past experiences, including having an abusive, alcoholic father, a heavily drinking mother and abusive experiences and relationships with men, the possibility of complex post-traumatic stress disorder (CPTSD) is indicated. This involves having been systematically abused and neglected, rather than experiencing a one-off traumatic experience, which is more relevant to PTSD, and recovering (Herman, 2015). The multiaxial DSM-V (APA, 2013) conceptualises post-traumatic stress disorder in a single broad diagnosis (Macneil et al., 2012), whereas the ICD-11 (World Health Organisation, 2019) details two disorders: PTSD and CPTSD. However, it is hoped to see the person beyond the diagnosis.

The question arises: To what extent is formulation an adequate alternative to psychiatry and whether a both/and approach is desirable or achievable (Cromby et al., 2013, p. 103)? Diagnosis can be very life-limiting. Perhaps, the diagnostic categories were intended as descriptive terms of patterns of symptoms for practice, where reliability and validity are irrelevant (Cromby et al., 2013, p. 111). Formulations possibly reframe diagnosed distress such as schizophrenia regarding trauma, abuse and bereavement using multi-perspectives (Weerasekera, 1996). Additionally, formulation appears to be a westernised construct, embedded in western assumptions, where greater cultural understanding of emotions is needed (Reddy, 2020).

Assessment is considered incompatible with the person-centred approach, according to Mearns. However, Joseph and Worsley (2005) advocate working with different approaches, such as psychometric assessments. According to Wilkins and Gill (2003, p. 183), person-centred practitioners engage in an initial process of information gathering within the contractual procedure; therefore, it is not the concept of assessment that is eschewed but its purpose to diagnose distress (Sanders, 2005).

Furthermore, 'Sandra's' mixed-race heritage requires attention regarding her possibly feeling powerless and threatened, with a father abusing her gender, relevant to the power-threat-meaning-framework (Johnstone & Boyle, 2018). 'Sandra' has no safe place to go to; in her accommodation, workmen intrude, possibly symbolising her perceived powerlessness. Perhaps if 'Sandra' tells the university about her experiences, she fears they may consider her unfit to work. This case study, perhaps, highlights the need for further work on cultural sensitivity in diagnostic terminology, alongside an evaluation of other aspects of the power-threat-meaning-framework in practice, using a range of methodologies (Johnstone et al., 2018, 2019, pp. 308–313), regarding patterns of distress (Johnstone et al., 2018).

Other social justice and inequality models facilitate working with 'Sandra's' genderised and racialised conditions of worth (Chantler, 2005). Bronfenbrenner's (1977) model, highlighted 'Sandra's' wider systems, reframing 'Sandra' within her sociocultural context, involving oppressions. Kegan et al.'s model (2011) highlighted 'Sandra's' right to self-determination, peacefulness, freedom and fair treatment. Goodman et al. (2004) add: consistent self-reflection, sharing resources, speaking out, increasing consciousness, strengths highlighted and equipping 'Sandra' with the skills for change, alongside deconstructing symptoms/diagnosis and collaborative/participatory formulation (McClelland, 2014).

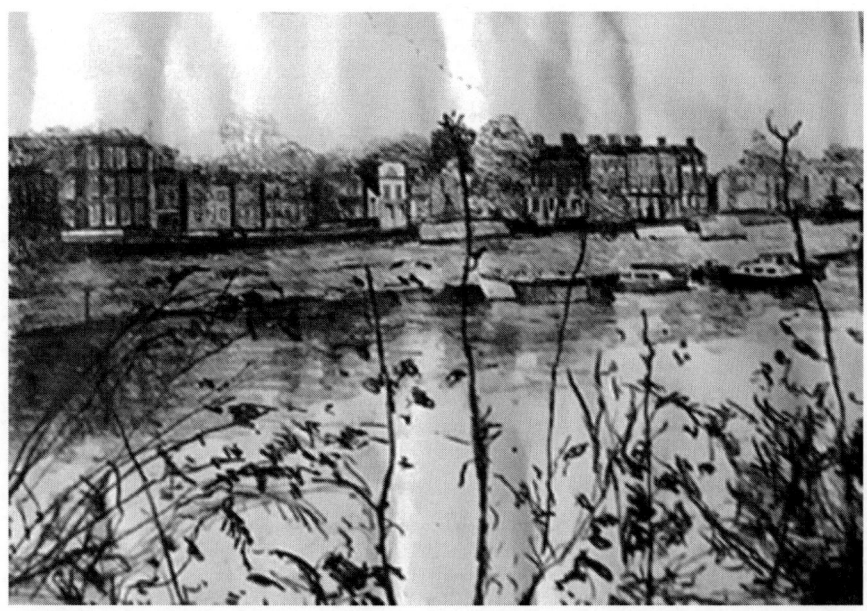

*Figure 7.2* Chiswick drawing

Regarding 'Sandra', having discussed the different therapy modalities, she declined sharing about herself in a group due to her vulnerability. We discussed several one-to-one therapeutic approaches and peer support, which were encouraged whilst waiting for a therapist. 'Sandra' preferred a longer-term psychotherapy with a female therapist. 'Sandra' was referred initially for a year for her directionality regarding her actualising tendency and for considering her as an 'integrated psycho-social-political whole' (Cooper, 2021, p. 6).

In summary, assessment and formulation are often significant markers for clients, and the limits require clarification. Rogers's work (1951, 1961a, 1992) supports collaborative assessment of the potential for a therapeutic relationship, embedded in Buber's 'I-Thou' vision (Buber, 1970). Psychometric tests can distract from the assessment relationship and client perspective but can facilitate shared dialogues, blending lived experiences with information. Risk can then be openly discussed, alongside diagnosis and medication queries. Focusing on the client's strengths and resources is advocated, alongside cultural considerations and client preferences in the therapy plan. The power-threat-meaning-framework is considered a helpful alternative to diagnosis, alongside the Simms's model (2011).

## Note

1 PHQ-9 is the nine-question depression scale from the Patient Health Questionnaire, GAD-7 is the Generalised Anxiety Disorder Questionnaire, and WSAS is the Work and Social Adjustment Scale used to assess client's perspective on 'impaired functioning'.

# 8    Case study 4 – 'Carlos' – a loss

'O, that this too too solid flesh would melt thaw and resolve itself into a dew! Or that the Everlasting had not fix'd His canon 'gainst self-slaughter!'

*Hamlet*, Act I, Scene II – William Shakespeare

## Carlos

'Carlos' was a handsome late 20-year-old mid-build male, who was sectioned on the acute ward, likely related to substance misuse and self-neglect. He was a brown-skinned, well-read and creative Italian but seemed directionless, alone and frightened, alongside being gifted and talented as an artist. It was on Carlos's second day on the ward when he and I met. Carlos appeared highly agitated and unable to recognise my presence, shaking and seeming very frightened, which made me aware of his vulnerability and that he was likely enduring a psychotic episode alongside trauma. The ward provisions were far from adequate, with only curtains separating one patient from another, which didn't take account of safety and privacy matters, in my opinion. Carlos had been brought to the ward by his father, who had informed Carlos that they were going to the park, but when Carlos recognised the route to the hospital, he jumped out of the car with his guitar. Carlos's father called the police due to his anxieties about his son's mental health and safety but needed to rush away to a business work meeting. It appeared that Carlos's father, Stephano, was rushed to get to his work meetings. Carlos's mental health was deprioritised, and he was abandoned with strangers – the police and hospital staff. It struck me that perhaps what was most needed for Carlos was his parents' consistent and reliable attention, understanding, love and care. On first meeting Carlos, it struck me how Carlos was shaking like a leaf throughout his whole body, face and speech. He seemed traumatised and terrified, trembling throughout his being. His hair was matted, and his expression was one of having given up in life, eyes turned down to the ground, disappointed with life, silenced by oppression, unloved, unappreciated, powerless, beaten down, ruined – tragic.

DOI: 10.4324/9781003509059-9

During the first few days of Carlos being on the ward, his younger sister, Serena, visited him and was pained to observe that Carlos appeared very distracted, particularly in regard to the squalid environment he was in. Carlos told his sister not to come and visit him for her sake, but she was adamant that she would stick by him: 'You are my brother. Of course, I will come and see you'. Serena travelled daily on her moped to visit Carlos, bringing food and drink for him, after college, where she was trying to undergo A levels, which Carlos had always been interested in. Carlos stated to Serena that he doesn't recognise his parents. As I had been asked to supervise visits to Carlos, I wondered if this was a comment on how he felt unrecognized and unacknowledged himself.

On the ward, Carlos shared a lot with me, often through trembling lips and shaking body, and I felt a river of tears in my countertransference. 'Perhaps the shaking managed his feelings of grief', I pondered to myself. He painted colourful, beautiful paintings and drew exact lifelike reflections of plants and views from the window, which were remarkably accurate. I wondered what was going on here, since his drawings indicated a clear, astute mind, yet he often spoke so abstractly that it was difficult to know what he meant, about shapes of words. For example, one morning with bright sunshine flooding through the hospital windows, he said to me:

The sun creates all kinds of shapes in my mind, which stops me from doing what I want to do. It's the shapes that are important to understand, it's the shape of things.

I was always interested to talk with individuals and strained my mind to come to realise what Carlos was communicating to me. Meeting with people like Carlos proved to be a profound experience in this 'holding' environment of crisis, of life and death. I offered that looking at the sun created shapes in my mind too. Carlos was quick to clarify that he thought that he knew what I meant but that he didn't mean sun specks but more in the mind. Try as I might to stretch my mind to understand what he meant, it was beyond me to grasp at the time, but I held my mind open to keep searching for Carlos's meaning so that I could connect more with him; he was strong enough to assert that he thought that I didn't know what he meant. I read about shapes being important in the thinking of individuals diagnosed with autism years later but, of course, could not check the accuracy of this. This idea has clearly stayed in my mind.

I recall how gentle Carlos was with other patients on the ward, sensitive, astute, appropriately jovial, profound, playful. A female patient, 'Marigold', who appeared frightened and vulnerable, was a black Caribbean-born woman in her fifties. She was guardedly quiet and paranoid in her demeanour. Carlos sang to her, making her smile and laugh, bringing her to sit with us. Then she went to the bathroom. It happened that when she returned to sit with

Carlos and me, I thought I would see how they would get on without me as a staff therapist there. Having established their relationship by way of to-and-for conversation, I took myself to the same bathroom from which Marigold had just returned. I was surprised to see a fresh large turd in the bathtub, which can only have been hers since I had not seen anyone else use the bathroom. It being 7:15 AM, and most of the ward were in their bedrooms. It was only over time through establishing and building trust with Marigold that I came to understand that she experienced seeing snakes coming out of the toilet which understandably terrified her, and so to protect herself, she had to use the bathtub instead.

I had heard some of the nurses scolding her, but I had not enquired what it was about but picked up that, naturally, the situation repeated itself. I learned again that being non-judgemental in these and most situations is very important, to withhold judgement. Over time, I helped Marigold use the toilet, which was a gradual but determined process of having established trust, talking through the situation and showing understanding. This helped her experience that she could, first of all, approach the toilet, sit on it with her clothes fully on and that nothing adverse would happen to her. Even when she saw snakes, they were not harmful towards her. Marigold was, at first, terrified. Many patients on wards experience terror when attempting to use the bathroom. For a plethora of reasons and without creating dependency and, therefore, being professionally and humanely boundaried, one can really show understanding without knowing all the detail of people's fears, which, in this instance and many others, are not easily immediately discernible, and therefore, a reflective, observant approach is necessary in order to be present and help the patient overcome their fears through consistency, patient persistency and reliability.

I also found many patients referring to seeing or imagining seeing snakes in one form or another. A man in his sixties from an African country imagined snakes exiting and entering his rectum with great distress involved. Another African woman in her thirties experienced snakes trying to enter her vagina when around other people.

On the ward, once I had returned from the bathroom, Carlos was playing his deliberately out-of-tune guitar to Marigold, who giggled and attended to her clothes and appearance obsessively. She appeared comfortable with Carlos, but within herself, her moods and thoughts appeared to be changing constantly. My impression was that Carlos was a harmless, sweet person who, for whatever reasons, found it difficult at times to communicate verbally with others on a level of abstraction, but many liked him.

In our one to ones where I tried to involve art making with Carlos, he shared that he considered his father shut down emotionally and his mother naive. I held these thoughts in mind and listened out for anything further he may have wanted to share, without my asking questions, which I had learned on wards (and off wards) are often experienced as intrusive. Carlos told me about a large underground burrow that he had dug in his parents' garden, where he would go and sit for 'peace of mind'. It sounded intriguing how he had managed to dig this and why, but I felt in my countertransference sad and concerned since it reminded me of a grave. It seemed that Carlos was trying to be separate from his parents. He was easy to like and a person who seemed ahead of his time but very alone and vulnerable. Carlos shared that his friend had helped him dig this hole. I wondered what his parents made of it or if they knew of it.

I had wondered if Carlos was on the autistic spectrum since, at night, he would flick a towel to switch the light on and off repeatedly, which may have been comforting or self-soothing. I noticed in my countertransference that this action drew my attention to him and then drew me to him physically to discover what was happening. I wondered what was being repeated and what Carlos wanted or needed if anything.

I observed Carlos wear his sister's purple school leggings at times, and when visiting one day, she told me that she had wondered where her leggings had gone. Carlos wore these with a dress over the top and walked on the ward quite confidently. Perhaps wearing such clothes, which is much more openly done now than in the past, was safer on the ward as he discovered his identity. I imagine that Carlos's parents may have been disapproving. Patients had shared with me that they came into hospital to be themselves, the only place that they could be without judgement, which interested me and I thought further about. It raised questions for me regarding why people find themselves on wards and what this environment permits them to talk about and try out in relation to their identity. One woman from Ghana shared with me that she went into a hospital voluntarily to go mad with the others. I spoke to Carlos with my usual respect; however, he was dressed, and I hoped that the continuity of relating would help him feel he was accepted by me.

Carlos returned to the ward several times, then was housed in a sheltered accommodation about three miles from where his parents lived. There seemed to be such a disconnect between how Carlos thought and how his parents related to him. However, there was a such a depth of love demonstrated by Carlos towards his father, who went into hospital for a physical operation, and Carlos stayed with him overnight to ensure that he was okay. I observed his parents' bringing food and spending time with Carlos but not really seeming to connect with him, which felt sad. It was as if they were in automatic mode asking the same questions but not really listening to the answers or being able to do much more than bring food, visit and leave; it was as if there was a poverty of meaning in the relationships. Carlos's siblings were loving of him but controlled by their parents and themselves confused by the situation and with their own losses.

One to one, Carlos and I explored his sexuality. It seemed that he was curious about gender and sexuality and open to sexual relationships with the opposite sex, and this felt natural to him. I felt very comfortable offering therapy to Carlos one to one, but some of his experiences that he recounted were disturbing. Carlos shared that he had felt violently pushed out of the family home by his father somehow and didn't feel welcome there but had struggled with these feelings for all of his teenage years. Carlos considered that his father saw him as a competitor for his mother's attention. Furthermore, Carlos had come into conflict with his father several times by growing marijuana in their garden, which the father had uprooted and thrown in the bin. Carlos, then a teenager, was deeply affected by this since his childhood friend from his home country, with whom he had practically lived with until the family moved when Carlos was 13 years old, seemed to represent Carlos's uprooting at this particularly sensitive age of becoming an adult. Carlos described a settled and fairly happy life in Italy, where he had a wide group of friends, which he also had where he moved to the UK. He was sociable, and people liked him. However, his life in Italy sounded very settled in the countryside, where everything was relatively safe and secure. Carlos described how he had observed his father falling in love with a next-door neighbour and had started an affair with her, which he thought continued for many years, explaining his father's absence when the family moved into a UK house, where the previous owner had been an alcoholic.

I enjoyed the therapy sessions with Carlos and wondered how he had been diagnosed with schizoaffective disorder and gained invaluable insights regarding the symptoms of neglect and family emotional dysregulation and paternal absence. There was an impression of the family being silenced, with one single voice – that of the father. This seemed to be a central problem, where Carlos's needs had been ignored. Additionally, there appeared to be violence and aggression emanating from the father, and Carlos described how, when he was 4–5 years old, his mother asked him to say to his father that the family needed him. As the father was leaving the family home again to attend another conference, Carlos sat on his father's foot and clung to his leg, saying, 'We need you here. Please stay', to which Carlos's father stamped his foot, hurting Carlos, who fell off upset and shocked since he had demonstrated love, and anger or rage was returned. Another example, which Carlos described to me, was when they were in the car on holiday and Carlos was carsick and crying, Carlos's father stopped the car and ordered him out and drove off. Carlos's father then returned. Another experience involved Carlos's father being responsible for taking Carlos to primary school when Carlos was around 6 years old. However, Carlos's father put him on the bus instead, and Carlos ended up 20 miles out and not at school. A stranger phoned the school, informing them that Carlos was on his own and disorientated but had recalled the name of his school.

Carlos shared about turning to cannabis when he moved to the UK to cope with his parents and his new home environment. He had been sent to a very rough state school, where drugs were flowing. He became addicted to many unprescribed drugs amongst a large group of friends. Carlos recounted being bullied since he stood out with a Northern accent. His father acted out aggression, and Carlos was very sensitive; his mother was naive, letting Carlos's friends enter into the home and do what they wanted, with no boundaries and, therefore, no safety. Carlos described sitting at the top of the family home's stairs having taken black bombers (part amphetamine, part ion-exchange resin for slow release) and seeing the people at his sister's party in the family home as 'little black people'. It seemed that no one was aware of his state of mind, which felt disquieting. Carlos recalled sitting in the family dining room with a tea towel on his head in the dark, with no one (apart from his mother and siblings) trying to approach him, but Carlos was mute. It sounded that Carlos had become mentally very unwell and that it was difficult for the parents (father absent) to know what to do. It seems that Carlos was left in this state for a long time.

Carlos's life continued in the community in the shared accommodation. His life had become more active, and he appeared more ordered in his thoughts, although still with matted hair. His sister had given him a black sparkly jumper, which he always wore, and I think he felt safe with her. He only talked to his sister in the family for the last four years of his life, he didn't talk to anyone else. He was painting and told me that he had made a kaleidoscope and looked up to the sun through it to see the myriad colours inside. I had never thought to make a kaleidoscope and was intrigued by this idea, which he managed to share with me. Carlos was sociable and invited me to see his 'snake trail', a series of paintings showing a snake's body in bright colours. The snake trail is of significance, as it may represent Carlos communicating that it was time for him to move on – shedding the skin of the past and emerging in a new form. It was as if family and staff were so used to Carlos being unwell that when he was becoming better and needed support to think about next steps, people seemed not to have time. The situation had not been managed properly; the staff at the sheltered accommodation were inexperienced, and the manager blurred boundaries, offering therapy to Carlos's sister and asking her to keep this confidential, as he gained hours for a counselling training.

Carlos's uncle attended a meeting where Carlos had expressed wanting to take his own life, but this didn't seem to be taken as seriously as it should have been. Carlos was given the freedom to be in the community. The last time that Carlos was known to be alive was when he went to the family home asking to speak with his father about moving on, who was on the telephone discussing business and had shouted at Carlos to wait, with which Carlos left the family home. Carlos's whereabouts was unknown, and his family became more and more anxious. Carlos's uncle waited at the family home, anticipating Carlos's return. Whilst Carlos's parents were on holiday, Carlos's uncle received the news of Carlos's death, his dead body found in a field.

This news came as a profound shock and devastation to this family. The chapel where the funeral was held was crammed with friends, family and staff, all shocked by Carlos's sudden death at his age of 26 years old. Ultimately, Carlos was a vulnerable adult in the care of the local authority at his time of death, when he had started to recover and had looked into the kaleidoscope in the hope of a brighter future, but was badly let down; nobody had acted to safeguard him when he clearly stated what was going on for him. As healthcare professionals, we need to act immediately in relation to what vulnerable people are telling us, about their life and the risks. Carlos was excited about how life was becoming for him, but there was no structure in place to help manage his suicidality, perhaps born of what he had lost and the mountain he felt he had to climb alone into the future.

# 9 Case study 5 – 'Luma' – a case of schizophrenia and P-OCD

**'Schizophrenia is a horrible, horrible, horrible illness' – 'Luma'**

Luma was an attractive black woman in her late twenties, who spoke to me on the acute female ward, requesting therapy for anxiety. She recounted assertively that she had a diagnosis of treatment-resistant paranoid schizophrenia and that she considered that she suffered from pedophilia obsessive-compulsive disorder (P-OCD). She managed to share with me that she had previously had therapy for a year, which she considered had helped a lot and that she valued the therapist's help. I suggested that we meet initially to see if she felt that she wanted to continue, careful to facilitate a sense of choice and autonomy rather than Luma feeling obliged in any way. There was a controlling aspect to Luma's approach of me, which may be assertive but I think spoke of her sense of powerlessness as a black woman with severe mental health difficulties in the UK.

## Background

Luma was born in another continent, where she excelled at school, describing being 'the top of the class'. Her mother suffered from schizophrenia and left the family home when Luma was four years old, the third of five children by her mother and father. Luma's father had met another woman, and one day, when Luma returned from school, she encountered her father in bed with her new step-mother. In this stark way, Luma was introduced to her step-mother. Luma's birth mother left the home very hurt, and Luma only saw her blood mother a few times over a 32-year period.

Luma shared with me that at her age of 8 years old, an aunt, 'Magdala', aged around 25 years old at the time, was assigned as Luma's surrogate mother and flew with her to Australia to see if another branch of her family would allow Luma to stay with them, but Luma reported how hostile they were towards her and Magdala. Subsequently, Magdala and Luma travelled to the UK, where they resided for the next 30 years. Magdala was given money by Luma's father for her upkeep, he was a wealthy businessman. Luma described some kind of affectionate bond with Magdala and how she had made sure

DOI: 10.4324/9781003509059-10

she ate and went to school but had been reportedly emotionally neglectful and what appeared to be abusive. Emotional neglect was described by Luma in terms of having no parental guidance about what to do or not to do, which she repeatedly bitterly regretted but had insight into. Magdala did not talk with Luma but did to her own blood child, which understandably was difficult for Luma, who considered that this deeply negatively impacted her self-esteem and sense of growth and development. An example of emotional abuse was recounted by Luma, who described Magdala talking on the phone to her friend about Luma, describing Luma in very derogatory terms, which affected her deeply and long-term.

Luma described going to school, but due to having no emotional support and left to her own devices, her school grades deteriorated as did her mental health. By the age of 18, Luma was seeing a boyfriend whom she loved and was sexually active in a mutually compatible relationship. However, when Luma was 22, she started hearing multiple intrusive voices and was found screaming in the street and was hospitalised. Magdala then had very little time for Luma, but Luma knew that she could turn to Magdala but that she may not help her. Luma became increasingly isolated from her family, most of whom were abroad and found it difficult to manage Luma's multiple phone calls and repeated highly personal and sensitive narratives, mainly about masturbation. It is important to note that Luma had managed to gain a degree and demonstrated resources. Luma was a very intelligent woman. Luma had been hospitalised due to being found screaming again in the street, and it was in a hospital that I met her on an acute ward. My memory recalls the following:

> Luma approached me slightly aggressively stating 'I asked for that word to be taken off my bedroom wall but no one has, it's really really disturbing me. I don't like the food here and I don't like the curtains in my room. This place has gone to ruin, the last time I was here it was really nice, I may discharge myself but I need my medication to be changed, my medication is making me highly sexually aroused but I am trying not to masturbate, anyway it's not private to do that here. I called my older brother today but he got annoyed said stop talking all that nonsense, all you talk about is masturbating and you repeat the same conversation, I don't have time for it. I was really upset since he is a great support to me. Can we talk somewhere private?' I said that we could, checked with the nurse in charge and indicated the one-to-one counselling room where we went. I asked Luma what she thinks she would talk about if she didn't talk about masturbation and she said about her early memory with her younger brother.

## Therapy with Luma

The ward consultant had approved me to work with Luma to help her feel heard about what was on her mind, if Luma found it helpful. I was very careful to detail the bounds of confidentiality, especially to try to instil some more consistent boundaries for Luma. Upon first meeting in the basic family room on the acute ward, I could see immediately that Luma held her integrity highly, which is rare to encounter in life. However, I hold Luma's sense of moral integrity in mind in relation to her sense of guilt which was a strong feature of her predicament. In the initial meeting, before I could blink, she had rushed ahead into the consulting room. I managed to get ahead of her so that she felt contained and so that I could be in the room with her to show her where to sit and take necessary charge of the therapy. It seemed that, with no consistent and reliable parental figure in her life, she was understandably uncontained, her Id unreined, in Freudian terms and impulsively rushing ahead – perhaps understandably and uncontrollably excited to have someone offering their time and attention for her.

I realised, through listening to Luma, that her sense of rushing into the counselling room was to quickly tell someone what was happening for her since she had been carrying it for so long and was terrified to tell anyone in case they thought that she was a pedophile. I recall her sitting on the edge of the ward couch; my mind was full of her impulsivity and childlike vulnerability and determination, Luma being very difficult to age. Luma was assertive, with attempts to manipulate me almost naively at times, and I considered this as a communication of her vulnerability and fear. I did not feel diminished by this in any way. I took the lead on talking through the working agreement so that she was aware of the terms and conditions, about which she read through carefully, rightly taking her time, and this was certainly encouraged by me, with plenty of space for her to raise any questions. Once signed, Luma and I could focus on the important aspect of what brought her to therapy, which Luma had, understandably, found it hard not to talk about on the ward, exposing herself further. I pay attention to the words used in turn to describe therapeutic situations, for example, why 'exposing herself' arises here. Luma stated that she deeply regretted sharing what she had on the ward, but it was important to put this into perspective and normalise the utterance she had made and think how to talk about what, where and when. Luma's potential lack of being held through her childhood and teens, with few limits set and a lack of interest shown in her, seemed to lead to impulsivity, which greatly interfered with relationships, leading to her isolation, abandonment and frustrations, which is very sad.

Luma was brave to come and speak with me, and I underestimate what it takes for an individual to reach a point where they can't hold it in any longer and have to take the risk of telling someone, which is by no means easy before, during or after such exchanges. I could see Luma bursting with anxiety and words, as she told me that she was masturbating many times due to what she had thought was her medication. She reported a great sense of relief at talking to me, like a weight was lifted from her. Luma had shown me the medication leaflet, which indeed referenced sexual arousal as a side effect. Luma spoke about her fears regarding when she masturbated that she heard children outside or on the TV, evoking anxieties of her being a pedophile. She was terrified that her masturbation was linked to children, although she never sought children out as a source of sexual gratification and was not in the least sexually attracted to children of any age. Luma and I discussed coincidence, but Luma was anxious that it may not be coincidental that when she masturbated, she heard a child's voice. In fact, as we worked together getting to know what was going on for her in relation to children, as she was out in the world or saw children on the TV, Luma reported being afraid of children who made her feel vulnerable. Luma appeared concerned in case she may have sexual feelings for children, but it was very clear to me that this was not the case. It may be that children evoke vulnerability in Luma, since when asked, she could not think of an adult who she could turn to when young.

Luma was additionally clearly extremely paranoid, and it felt like her mind was trapped in a horror film where the reel replayed daily, communicating to me about her life currently – insecure, alone and unsafe. I learned to trust Luma's perception on most matters alongside questioning what she said; her assessment of people seemed particularly astute during the course of the therapy. My genuine sense of trust in her perceptions and thoughts helped her to feel that she could trust herself. I communicated that I was aware of the pros and cons of the mental health system, which she commented helped her feel more at ease. Luma shared that she was part of a community mental health team but that she had had to informally admit herself in the past to reduce her medication.

Luma and I discussed her current situation, an important aspect of which involved discussing in detail about her fears of being sexually attracted to children, which she was consistently clear that she was not. I checked this out in various ways, enquiring about her bodily sensations when she was with children, and it was clear that she had no sexual thoughts or interest in children of any age and Luma agreed. I had worked with others who had almost exactly the same fears about children, and I helped normalise anxieties with reference to P-OCD being a recognised condition. I think that this developmental phase may be far more common than is understandably discussed and therefore known. I wondered about why Luma thrust masturbation so heartily into the forefront of discussions and what may be underpinning this. Luma was increasingly cooperative in relation to the therapeutic process; she valued integrity, but I also considered her possible scrupulosity as a possible aspect of Luma's OCD traits and in relation to her religiosity, which was relevant to her. Luma was very able to build a therapeutic relationship with me based on trust. I was moved that she had a relationship with another whom she trusted, which I hoped would be a protective factor for her. I encouraged her to establish and form as many relationships as possible, as people for her to turn to and to replace the family she did not have in the UK.

Then Luma openly shared a sensitive childhood experience, recollected from her age of around 6 years old. Luma recalled having been in a room with her baby brother, around his age of 1 year old. She recalled that her brother was lying on the floor below the closed window; she recalled starting to lift her dress with the intention of placing one foot on either side of her brother's body to 'jump up and down on his privates'. On further exploration, Luma was not sure how she would have done this but stated that she never intended to go any further. Luma expressed curiosity from when she was aged 6 about her brother's sexuality. Luma recalls her aunt entering the room, arms folded, giving her 'a stern look', and Luma knew that it was wrong what she was about to do and stopped. Luma shared with me that through her aunt's stern look, Luma thought the aunt knew what she was about to do. Luma stated that 'God knows what would have happened if she had not come in' and how this would have left Luma, living with that now. Luma spoke of just about being able to assuage herself since she had not acted on what she considered to have been her intention. Luma found it understandably difficult to think about this memory, able to decrease her sense of guilt by reminding herself that she was a child then. Luma and I discussed this situation in some detail, and she would tell me that she did not want to talk about it any further, which I respected.

Through supervision, it was considered therapeutic to try to explore with Luma this childhood experience. Luma and I wondered why she was alone in a room with her 1-year-old brother and that the theme of a lack of parental guidance may be relevant at this early age, when her blood mother had left the family home and was suffering with schizophrenia. The status of this memory was also thought about in terms of a possible screen memory at a point in Luma's life inaccessible to her or denied. Luma stated that she had never been violated sexually by anyone in her family. She had, however, thought for many years that an uncle had interfered with her, recalling him sleeping with her in the same bed and lifting her above his head when she was around the age of 8 years old. Luma considered now that he had not done anything to her.

In supervision, Luma's communications were discussed anonymously. Supervision considered that the early childhood experience was the difficulty that needed addressing in the present and that the masturbation content distracted from other more painful issues. I tended to agree with this since Luma had her accounts of masturbation to bring to me too readily and would fill the whole session if I allowed it; Luma was retelling her narrative to correct it obsessively. I noted that Breuer and Freud (1895) mention masturbation with furniture in their *Studies on Hysteria*. Luma had similarly recounted to me instances of having masturbated with furniture through her childhood, adolescence and adulthood, now reportedly stopped. On one occasion, Luma had masturbated with furniture with a female cousin who had eventually left before Luma had wanted to lay on top of her. On another occasion, Luma had been observed by a family member, and this had been spread around many, much to Luma's embarrassment and shame.

My understanding of my role as therapist is not to offer reassurance to clients since this most often is false and, therefore, potentially misleading.

However, Luma and I were able to go back to the basics and agree that she was not sexually attracted to children at any point in her life but perhaps angry at her brother's new presence (sibling rivalry), and this possibly led to aggressive thoughts towards him, alongside curiosity about his sexuality. When in her home country growing up, she had been comfortable with children in the family and had shared with me that, on one occasion, she was happy to jump out of a window when she thought that a child may have come to harm. This, of course, raised concerns for me, but Luma explained that this demonstrated the degree of her care to avoid harm to children.

I felt that I got to know Luma, as she attended every ward therapy session on time and was open to sharing with me, perhaps partly due to my concerted efforts to establish and maintain a consistent and reliable working therapeutic relationship, where she felt supported and not judged, she feedback to me. It seemed to me, and as discussed in supervision, that Luma was a fairly dominant personality and a leader, perhaps partly due to her brightness but also that she may have had to manage herself from an early age and hence develop faster than her chronological age. I often was confused by her age. In subsequent therapy sessions, Luma and I worked through her guilt, which was often avoided by talking about her familiar subject of masturbation, which she strongly believed was due to the medication. Although painful, having established and maintained such a strong working alliance with Luma, she was able to face the early experience with her brother at her age of 6 years old. This work required skill and persistence to work it through, or this core memory may have remained intact with its repeating emotional reverberations. Luma and I explored her sense of guilt and wish to avoid the experience. Additionally, Luma and I discussed how she felt around children in everyday life, which greatly reduced her anxieties, and she was more at ease with her thoughts of being with children, gaining strength from the security and safety of our working alliance.

By session nine, Luma wanted to progress more, eager to learn something new about herself. She was friendly, respectful, humorous and insightful, eager to make something of herself yet finding herself in a mental health system that struggled to move her life on for her. I was impressed with Luma's insight to withdraw from a medication to find out if the sexual arousal she spoke of so frequently was due to the medication or to her hormones, as she also pondered being possible. I felt that Luma's need to repeat her accounts of masturbation and then repeat and correct were related to her fear that I could not hold what she said in mind, alongside a need for perfection and her deprivation and early sexual experiences not yet recollected. Luma and I discussed what she was spending her life doing: stating, correcting and restating repeatedly what she had done. I asked her what she would think about if she didn't recount these narratives, and she said that she would think about getting a job, using her degree and finding a boyfriend. Luma's paranoia became reportedly so intense two to three times daily that she could not function with looking after herself, and she often spoke about wanting to die. She found London oppressive and, at every turn, a reason to make money. Luma felt understandably suicidal. The government in power at the time left so many feeling similarly totally hopeless.

I used all of my skills possible, discussing different situations, triggers, thoughts and images. Luma shared that she often felt anxiety in relation to thinking about the past and future and often was having a bad day (paranoid) and feeling angry, hurt and upset about her paranoia and the medication side effects described as 'episodes' by her. Luma discussed her feelings further, mainly of fear and sadness but also disgust at herself and feeling fearful, frightened and anxious. Luma further described feelings of vulnerability, stress, frustration and panic. Her main fearful thought was that she was going to kill herself or someone else out of anger and frustration. Luma had deeply self-harmed when paranoid, and a policeman entered into her home and read her diary, despite her telling him not to. Another major fear from Luma was that when masturbating, a voice spoke, 'sex with children', and again, the timing evoked anxiety for her, alongside doubt that she may be a pedophile. She reported having no images at such times but was aware of fearing telling someone else about what was happening for her. Eventually, Luma did feel more in control to talk to her care coordinator about more of her experiences, which brought its consequences since she then regretted what she had shared, feeling exposed and fearful as to with whom this information would be shared and notes written. Luma and I explored facts, providing evidence against the unhelpful thought that she may kill herself or someone else, that she was still alive and wanted to be alive. We discussed how her fear of killing herself provided further evidence that she didn't want to kill herself and had never tried to or killed anyone in the past. Then Luma and I explored an alternative, more realistic and balanced perspective whereby Luma thought that she was angry and didn't know how to express it. Upon further exploration, Luma stated that she was angry about having schizophrenia and that it seemed never-ending, alongside being angry that she felt lonely and anxious (cognitive-behavioural therapy approach – thought records at Luma's request).

At Luma's request, she and I underwent a collaborative assessment of possible vicious cycles in her life to clarify what was maintaining her difficulties. Luma brought her own well-thought-out vicious cycle on paper to the next therapy session. Luma explained that her anger was linked to intrusive thoughts, images, urges and doubt, where the meaning was that having this thought meant that I may act on it or that she was in danger of it happening. Luma described thinking biases, for example, catastrophic thinking, which leads to avoidance and safety-seeking behaviours, such as mental reassurance and checking. Luma identified her feelings as fear and disgust. Her disgust was at herself for her thought towards her brother when she was 6 years old.

I encouraged Luma to take her leave from the hospital ward to gain from fresh air and exercise. I also considered it helpful for her to deliberately go out and be where children were and to notice her thoughts, feelings, bodily sensations and behaviours. It became clear that Luma remained frightened of children in relation to triggering her fears about her potential pedophilia. For example, Luma was afraid of looking up children on the internet in her sleep, then locking her phone in a drawer but still fearing what she may do in her sleep. Luma and I worked through the logic of emotion to think through what she was most afraid of, how likely the feared event was to happen and what would happen if it did. Luma was hungry to trust and gain help and her exponential suffering was difficult yet possible for me to think about, but I needed to know my limits whilst trying everything I could to help her. Luma was reticent to discuss her religiosity because she thought that I would like her less, which was nowhere in my thinking but indicated how she felt threat externally. Her feelings of shame and guilt appeared to find expression through religiosity, and we talked openly in exploring such difficult thoughts and feelings. I came to think that Luma's low self-esteem was a consequence of her surrogate mother publicly shaming her and blaming her without any attempts to understand why the situations had arisen and her surrogate mother's part in the situation.

I wondered with Luma what she was looking for in a hospital, and she said respite, to be looked after and to feel safe. She discharged herself, finding the ward consultant aggressive and bullying, yet she was able to stand her ground and maintain her boundaries of confidentiality when he enquired about her personal relationships and their names. However, weeks later, Luma felt it necessary to readmit herself to gain a further medication reduction, which the care coordinator would not progress for her otherwise.

I had managed the transition from inpatient therapy to private therapy, mostly due to Luma's facilitation of this and trust in our working relationship. The ward consultant helpfully facilitated this move. CMHT staff tried to gain access to speak with me, in private practice, without Luma's consent, which I was not willing to go ahead with and felt concerned that they posed this to me, putting me under pressure to agree to do so. When I detailed the terms of confidentiality to Luma at the start of therapy, I meant what I said.

It was heartening how much Luma could think between therapy sessions. She turned up to the next sessions and announced that she wanted to visit her home country, where the majority of her family were – father, step-mother, sisters, aunts, brothers, half-siblings and mother. This immediately felt right and made sense to me for her to go and be amongst her family since her life was isolated and meaningless in the UK. Her quality of life was very limited and her suffering immense, often including suicidal thoughts and one incident of severe self-harm to hold in mind. Luma and I weighed up the pros and cons and thought about her housing and how to manage it with a plan. We discussed her finances and whether she could afford to pay for a single or return flight. Once such discussions had progressed and Luma had bought a return ticket, we spent a lot of time planning her approach to the airport,

Luma and I psychically walking through customs due to the paranoia and a detailed examination of what this may trigger for her and how to manage it.

I helped her think about how to behave and respond, and all eventualities were covered. Luma was understandably very frightened about making this move and about whether she would manage the journey to her family. Luma and I discussed this in many sessions before she was due to fly. All practicalities were thought about and discussed in detail with her, with a plan for each. She picked up her medication to take with her and a letter from the CMHT stating that her diagnosis had been reduced from treatment-resistant paranoid schizophrenia to schizoaffective disorder, which she was very pleased about. Her friend accompanied her to the airport, which Luma and I had discussed. Luma successfully navigated customs and the flight, then meeting with her father for the first time in 11 years was very moving to read about in her text, confirming her arrival there. I felt that she had made a great achievement, and I was very happy for her. I was also mindful of how her family would treat her, which she and I had discussed.

Luma requested therapy whilst abroad, and she took up this offer, again discussing her housing and wish to return to the UK. Luma was making good progress in her family, feeling stronger. Luma's medication had been reviewed and stopped, yet she still experienced high sexual arousal, clarifying that this was not linked to the medication. Luma reported two further medications being stopped, radical moves compared to the UK. I think about how she is getting on with her family and hope that she is moving towards fulfilling her several constructive aims: get a job, find a boyfriend to marry and possibly have children and to be happy.

Thinking about Luma, within six months, she had been able to grow enough in the therapy to face her isolated state. Why she was really in the UK remains a mystery, and being separated from her parents, brothers and sisters from the age of 8 years old is painful. Her suffering was immense, and she talked to me about her upbringing – lack of parental guidance being at the root of her diagnosis. I think that with the right, consistent and reliable care and attention, she would gradually flourish. It seems to be her sense of self through neglect, abuse and abandonment that has pushed her mind out of reality, likely to manage the cruel reality she would otherwise face. Luma thanked me for all my help. She said she was glad to see the back of this country with all its rules for money and red tape, stating then that she never wanted to return. Luma sadly felt like a second-class citizen in the UK, but I hope that I returned a sense of dignity to her life. Since then, the UK have had a successful election, and life in the UK seemed less turbulent.

Luma has asked for more online therapy whilst abroad, and she spoke about how she had been taken off all her medications and hospitalised through this process. Luma now is on two medications only and sounds like a different person on the call, sounding clearer and more coherent, yet I hold this update with caution since it is easy to think that all is cured, from my own unconscious hopes. Luma shared about feeling torn between mothers and missing her aunt in the UK, where she had been raised for 30 years. I interpreted that perhaps Luma has a stable reference point with her aunt in the UK, alongside her 'good therapist', whom she wanted to see 'as soon as I get back'. I thought that this raised a question for Luma about who she is and where she belongs. Luma has experienced unstable parenting and sadly has introjected an unstable internal world subsequently, with little clarity about who her basic relatives are. These fundamental questions would evoke uncertainty and anxiety for her. I discussed in supervision about interpreting her anxieties in the transference, exploring whether she has a good sense of who she is. My supervisor considered that I am a stable reference point for Luma, noting that she has good contact with me. He also suggested enquiring with Luma about how she considers me, what makes her feel who she is and who the important references are for her.

In relation to this anxiety, Luma shared with me that she felt torn between her mothers and their religions, which felt very difficult for her and for me managing the situation thousands of miles away. I felt concerned that Luma had severely self-harmed in the past. I was aware that Luma had felt suicidal on a daily basis but didn't want to act on this, alongside having thoughts to kill or harm others due to her frustration, depravation and anger. I was unsure how the emergency services worked where she was. It is clear that throughout the therapy in the UK and support abroad, Luma was motivated to gain a better life, the original reason why she had come to the UK at her age of 8 years old. Luma had informally admitted herself to a hospital to reduce her medication to try to alleviate her sexual arousal and travelled to her family for a better life opportunity, managing to progress reconvening with her family and a significant medication review. She had given up smoking abroad, leading to a need to increase her clozapine before it was eliminated.

From abroad, Luma shared that the electricity came and went and that this was disruptive to life. I interpreted with Luma that it was difficult for her to function as a person with her current internal world, like the lights and electricity going on and off. I observed a healthy side and a confused side to Luma, the confused part intruding a lot on the healthy side, who wants a better life – job and marriage with children. I considered in supervision how a boyfriend (Luma had stated that she 'wants' to be heterosexual due to her religion) would be important in relation to her sexual issues and driven sexual impulses in her sexual organs and have a stable person to feel stable within herself regarding her very difficult, frequent, multi-daily, paranoid episodes. It is especially important for Luma and others in a similar situation that I remain a benign authority as an internal stabilising object inside herself and to be aware that this state can descend into a paranoid state. It seems Luma's paranoia can erupt from nowhere, perhaps linked to her aunt's comments about her.

Luma's paranoia showed itself in relation to her thinking that the TV was talking to her and instructing her to masturbate in front of it, which she managed, via the ritual of saying her ex-boyfriend's name for protection, since she feared harmful incidents happening to her otherwise. Luma feared that when she felt instructed by voices in her mind to masturbate in front of the TV and that if she, by chance, heard a child's voice on the stairs outside her flat, this indicated that she was a pedophile. Luma and I returned to the question of whether she was sexually attracted to children, which she consistently responded to in the negative. I was aware that Luma saw me supporting her abroad on a screen when she was in therapy with me, and I wondered how can she gain a clear distinction between what was actually on the TV screen and with the online screen with me on it too. I sought to help Luma with distinguishing different realities, at first totally convinced that the TV was instructing her to masturbate, and further on in therapy, Luma was able to consider the possibility of this not being the case. Such movements for Luma and the therapy are moving and significant, showing that with moment-to-moment observation and careful intervention, change can happen. I felt that Luma learned well in therapy, contradicting traditional views that individuals with psychosis can't be helped. Therapy appeared as a pathway towards sanity for Luma, or the TV would talk to her with psychotic presence. Luma wanting to return to the UK, I held in mind as a possible impulse to see me as a consistent external object, even if she hasn't currently got an internal stable object in her mind.

Luma shared about wanting to find a man to marry and have children with. I considered that she wanted to find a love object in her genitals and her mind to find internal satisfaction and help her feel she has an identity, rather than being damaged goods, despite her stepsister's mother's comment. I think that in Luma saying that her family abroad cannot sustain her needs, for example, her healthcare costs, she appears to be wondering who can help her to be with herself somehow. Perhaps this is the motivation to move back to the UK and to link up with objects to help her know what she is thinking. Luma spoke often of her male friend who visited her in the UK five times a week and was physically overly friendly, but Luma may well feel desperate for presence to reassure her through her terrifying paranoid experiences. Luma greatly valued this friendship, whom she considered her best friend. Luma appears to be seeking stability (external scaffolding): a job and boyfriend, seen as stabilising influences.

When Luma regularly repeated narratives of her masturbatory experiences, she needed to retell the story to correct what she considered were errors, trying to perfect something that could not be perfected and worrying greatly about the mistakes, compulsively repeating what seemed to be screen narratives of the memory when she was 6–7 years old with her 1-year-old brother. I considered the transference regarding my presence in her mind and her wanting to keep me external, possibly due to her unstable internal world, like a paranoid whirlpool or cesspit. I further considered how individuals with psychosis are anxious about internalising objects. If she is to gain some kind of stability in her mind, how can she internalise that and experience a person's presence when she is not with them and alone in her flat, for example? Luma didn't think that I would be thinking of her between sessions. She appeared genuinely shocked by this. However, Luma needed me in her mind, linked with her paranoid states, when no one was there when needed and only the TV screen to attack her.

My supervisor encouraged me to work towards considering her paranoid state as linked to her sense of self as an evil pedophile, as if her mind can get with a state as damaged as herself, or damaging towards others. I observed Luma, who seems to be one of the most honest people I have ever met, worrying about herself as displaying evil, damaged behaviour, which so easily took over her mind. To help her, perhaps she thinks that she must get back to her good therapist in the UK to reassure her that there is good in the world rather than a disastrous state of mind. Luma appeared lost in the instability between good and evil. Her brother told her to stop talking nonsense about masturbation; perhaps he felt there was something intolerable about this. I heard about Luma's masturbation a lot, and it was quite a fixed subject. Listening to her attempts to struggle with evil to get with an accurate, stable picture may be impossible to do. Luma's instability easily turned to evil, like evil was inside her in her genitals, representing her mind – a masturbatory mind in what appeared to be an infantile, primitive state.

# 10   Case study 6 – 'Melanie'

To weep is to make less the depth of grief:
Tears then for babes; blows and revenge for me.
Henry VI, Part III, Act II, Scene I

My work with 'Melanie' constitutes one of my main therapeutic investments and professional learning experiences, with a woman of then 32 years old, now 47 years old following 15 years of frequent, weekly supportive therapy with me. Melanie had a diagnosis of paranoid schizophrenia, now an anxiety disorder with brief psychotic episodes. It is hard to describe how moving and fulfilling it is for me to hear of a reduced psychiatric diagnosis for Melanie in relation to her improved quality of life. My approach has been supportive and increasingly psychoanalytic as Melanie's fragility gradually turned to strength. I hope that this inadequate summary of my work with Melanie encourages others to take the time to make space for these suffering souls, who I think are crying out for understanding and can be helped.

## Background

At the start of therapy, Melanie was a 32-year-old black African woman whom I was assigned to as a therapist on an all-female acute ward by the ward consultant psychiatrist. Melanie was very concerned about her physical looks and wore a variety of wigs, which fascinated me and the cultural difference this highlighted between us. Her dress was very glamorous with long flowing white silk garments, perhaps as if she was about to attend an evening dinner party, or a wedding.

I wondered how our cultural differences may hinder communication, but Melanie was eager to communicate with me and overcome any obstacles on the way, perhaps, understandably very hungry to talk and be heard, lonely and isolated from her family and the world, who had abandoned her to some extent, as her father had left the family when she was young. She talked to me about her beliefs in black magic from her home country, which was of

DOI: 10.4324/9781003509059-11

immense interest to me. Melanie, having managed to gain a degree in social sciences, conversed eloquently regarding a range of topics. When I first met Melanie, she was heavily pregnant by eight months, reportedly by a man who had paid her money for a baby on the internet, which Melanie reported that she had done many times before. Despite her diagnosis of paranoid schizophrenia, Melanie was not prescribed any medication with concerns from the ward doctors about how this may affect her baby. It was planned that as soon as Melanie would give birth that her baby would be offered for fostering and adoption.

Part of my work with her was to work through her understandably very strong feelings about this, despite the decision having already been made by the multi-disciplinary team due to safeguarding on the grounds of her mental health, which Melanie also agreed with at the time. Melanie shared with me on the maternity ward, after she had given birth, that she realised that she wouldn't be able to cope with a baby at that point in her life. A further aspect of my therapeutic work with Melanie was to work with her family, who were very helpful in relation to informing me, with Melanie's consent, about her background from their perspective, creating a fuller picture and, with greater understanding, allowing me to think how best to help her.

Melanie had three sisters, one with whom she was still in contact; the other two had withdrawn their contact with Melanie due to her reportedly arriving at their homes at 3 AM and screaming outside to be let in, then pounding the door until she was let in. Melanie sounded to be very distressed at these times. I wondered about her distress and wanted to help her. 'Eleanor', her younger sister by two years, appeared older than Melanie, and this perhaps spoke of Melanie's needs being arrested at a certain age, perhaps preventing her fully developing emotionally. Eleonor shared with me when we met on the ward and spoke in a private family room that Melanie had, from an early age of 8 years old, been found wandering at night in her pyjamas and had to be brought home. Her father, with whom Melanie states she was close, left her mother when Melanie was aged 7 and had been very cruel to Melanie's mother, then left to move to his home country in Africa. At the age of 7 years old, Melanie states that she was raped in a local park and came home very distressed, but her father had gone, and her mother screamed, shouted at her and hit her violently.

Melanie's mother visited Melanie on the ward and agreed to speak with me again with Melanie's consent. Melanie's mother, 'Alvita', was of African-Caribbean ethnicity. She spoke to Melanie as if she was 5 years old, which may account for Melanie's part arrested development. Melanie was completely compliant in relation to her mother, which I have observed in other mother-daughter relationships, where the daughter experiences psychosis, as in the case study of Aasiya, in this volume. Both Melanie and Aasiya were, therefore, compliant, saying what pleased their mothers, who appeared harsh and undermining of their daughters. Melanie's mother, Alvita, had nothing positive to say about Melanie and spoke in a thought-disordered manner. I observed Alvita speaking mostly cruelly towards Melanie, and I intervened to prevent further harm being caused due to Melanie's vulnerable psychotic state of mind and her pregnancy. There were safeguarding concerns raised by me about Alvita, which added to the already documented record about her.

## Therapeutic work with Melanie

The ward consultant offered me weekly supervision for my therapeutic work with Melanie on the ward but didn't give me much information by way of background. I also benefited from fortnightly supervision with Professor Robert Hinshelwood. I wasn't given access to Melanie's medical notes, which is not my way of working generally speaking. I consider that having as much information as possible is informative regarding the individual's sensitivities and cultural background. Reading notes and letters helps gain a bigger picture, alongside querying the referral and what is being written into this person's presentation by the staff – the problem of the referring person (Palazolli et al., 1980). As professionals, we need to be much more alert and questioning of what is written about patients and staff for that matter.

Melanie and I discussed the issues that were arising in her life on the ward currently. In my countertransference, I felt acute violence in relation to meeting with Melanie one to one, which was terrifying in the moment, until reflecting that this was inside Melanie at the moment, but as I was aware of acute wards, feelings can very quickly become actions. I reflected on this acute feeling of violence and started to unravel complexities around, for example, her father leaving, Melanie being raped in the park, her mother's harsh contempt and neglect of Melanie and her schizophrenia, medication, intelligence, sisters, loss of life and pregnancy. Melanie was fully coherent and strong-minded most of the time, finding a solicitor to represent her regarding maintaining custody of her unborn child, which she gained. In order to safeguard the unborn child, the psychiatric team upheld that she may have custody of her child once born. They communicated to me that Melanie's newborn child would be referred for fostering and adoption, and Melanie immediately administered anti-psychotic and other medications. I felt ambivalent about this situation. Fortunately, Melanie's lawyer was straightforward with her, informing her that it was highly unlikely that she would have custody, but as Melanie processed this very difficult situation in her therapy with me, she was determined to fight for contact with her child, which I supported. Melanie showed me photos of ten or eleven other babies that she had, whose pictures she stuck on her bedroom wall in her flat. Melanie referred to her children a lot. The situation felt that Melanie needed to take responsibility for her problems and be in her skin rather than handing it over to others since she would be very angry at the staff, who were trying to help, speaking to them in a similar manner as her mother spoke to her. In therapy, I tried to help set boundaries with Melanie to protect her. I wondered in supervision whether Melanie was trying to move on from the abused child by having babies. It felt like Melanie was sharing a lot about her life and asking me to gather the bits together for her, which I would do as a therapist, mirroring a child-parent relationship.

It was extremely helpful that I had gained experience working on acute wards and working therapeutically with the patients on the wards. I was sensitive to their needs and able to read beyond how patients on acute wards were likely feeling, alongside establishing and developing a relationship with the more normal aspect of the personality. Additionally, I had an overview of the systems involved and experience of their strengths and areas for improvement. Melanie continued to share openly with me since I had put a lot of thought into clearly defining the boundaries of confidentiality. It is wholly unethical for therapists or other staff working with paranoid patients who are extremely vulnerable and often in crisis and, therefore, frightened and dependent, to have staff claiming confidentiality, then holding secret conversations where information is shared but without the patient's consent and then justifying this by GDPR. Melanie informed me that she had become pregnant through meeting someone once from the internet but had been paid £500 by the father to become pregnant and carry the baby, with the plan being to hand over the baby to the father once born. Melanie claimed that she had done this numerous times before and showed me photographs of her bedroom in her London flat strewn with babies' photographs, all of whom she stated convincingly that she loved very much but had had to let go of by giving them to men. I discussed with Melanie that I would need to raise this as a safeguarding concern, which I am unclear she understood or perhaps agreed with, but I documented our conversations and sent these to the safeguarding lead in the NHS Trust, where my work with Melanie was based. Restrictions were placed on Melanie's IT use on the ward, and we discussed her feelings about this and other aspects in her weekly ward-based therapy. Going to Melanie's flat with her as part of a discharge plan as the birth of her child drew nearer raised questions about how the transference and countertransference in the therapeutic relationship might make this very difficult. I also needed to consider my own safety.

When the time came for Melanie to be admitted to the nearest maternity ward, she asked me if I would attend the next day when she thought that she would give birth. The ward consultant approved this since she didn't really have anyone else, apart from her sister, who had her best interests at heart but wouldn't be attending for the birth. I attended on the ward after her birth and supported Melanie, who was tired and medicated, as planned by the mental health team. Melanie stated that she was happy to have given birth and that she was aware that her daughter would be given to a foster family. She understood that this was the best plan since she would not be in a position to take enough care of her. She said that as soon as she had given birth, her baby was taken into another room and that Melanie had been given a photograph of her, which she showed to me. Melanie's mother appeared and I noticed was pleasant to Melanie until she took the photograph of the newborn and disappeared with it from the ward.

Melanie asked me to go and meet her baby; she wanted me to meet her. I asked the nurse if this was okay, and they directed me to her, a tiny baby lying in a pram in a room where there were around ten other babies sleeping. I was surprised that there was no one with her. She was awake and reached out her tiny hand to me. I offered her my forefinger in relation to her size, and she grabbed it and started crying. It was very moving thinking that I would never see this life again and wished her well for the future, as a range of feelings flooded into my mind. My maternal feelings made me want to pick her up and at least hug her. I refrained from doing so, but to this day. I stayed with her for 20 minutes or so, with no one present in the room. I asked the nurses if anyone was offering her attention and comfort; she seemed utterly abandoned. The nurses stated that they would pay her attention, but when I left, there was no one with her.

I considered how feelings may get shut down by the sheer vulnerability of babies in such circumstances, perhaps under the premise that if they are being moved to a foster home, then it's best not to intervene. I strongly disagree with this and will never forget the degree of abandonment that these babies were experiencing in their first hours of life. I can only imagine the neglect occurring in different circumstances around the world, where our own infantile experiences become enacted in these highly charged situations. I have continued to wonder how this little girl is; she would now be 15 years old and had had such a difficult start in life. On the other hand, perhaps she is absolutely fine.

After Melanie's medication had settled in the next few weeks as she stayed on the ward for observation, her daughter was referred to a foster home quickly, but Melanie fought and gained contact with her, then saw her regularly, which was going well and was increased.

These therapy sessions were very difficult due to Melanie trying to manage her feelings of anxiety and rage about losing her baby. I empathised with Melanie about how I thought she may be feeling, but on reflection, I think that I was trying to persuade her that the sessions were safe, when, in fact, Melanie was likely anxious about hitting me in the one to one and avoided this situation, potentially feeling paranoid towards me. I veered away from saying anything analytic and said, 'I think you feel anxious', in order to be more realistic. In hindsight, I further think that it was not safe for me to be alone in a room with Melanie at this time since she appeared grandiose, and I became aware that it was important how I adapted to her rather than impose what is analytic. I acknowledged her rage in the context of a narrative of loss, as an attempt to meet her at her level, whilst thinking about the baby and mother in this exchange, feeling jarring for her in my countertransference. Melanie, perhaps, protected me from her violence by making me the good mother. I was very careful of such a transference since it could break down at any moment with explosive feelings for individuals with psychosis. Such strong feelings can be mind-blowing; they destroy the part of the ego that they can't stand – reality (Bion). They unconsciously destroy a capacity of perceiving reality and hallucinate to make up a reality in a non-reality form.

It can be thought that babies may well get into a state of wanting to be physically violent if they could be. It may be the infant part of Melanie emerging, recollective perhaps of her mother, who may not have been able to manage non-verbal holding, or to find words. I wondered if I had seen a possible crisis of rage and fear at what her perceived mother could do to her. Once I had conveyed to her that she had her own thoughts and was her own person and separate, Melanie then appeared to get into a paranoid state of being on her own, where she felt that no one was looking after her. Perhaps being separate was too much, and she may have felt abandoned as a result, then feeling critical in conflict, ambivalent. It seemed possible that being on her own was an assault on her existence; she knows that she is separate as an adult. However, a conflict emerges that she doesn't separate and gets herself into the ward, where she is looked after. There appears an oscillation, whereby if she has her own thoughts and feelings, she is going to have to cope with paranoid anxieties – the paranoia of mother after having her own feelings and own life. She can possibly feel pride, but she feels abandoned. Perhaps the adult grows, but the infant feels she is being trashed by another, who should merge with her and look after her. It seemed that Melanie may have had a phantasy of creating a boundary between a more independent part of herself and a part that would destroy everything, while also feeling vulnerable to being destroyed by the world, as described by Bion's understanding of the psychotic and non-psychotic parts of the personality. I was very careful about making verbal interpretations and veered towards reflecting back to Melanie about who was interested in her and who was willing to listen. In supervision, Professor Robert Hinshelwood considered that I should feel encouraged by my work with Melanie.

Melanie and I processed some very difficult feelings, bringing me a sense of sadness in my countertransference; Melanie was grieving a great deal, but this was not obvious from what I saw. Such unconscious communications of grief are essential for understanding what needs to be processed for the patient. Melanie became relatively stable in her mental state over the next few weeks, and it was planned for her to be discharged. The ward consultant asked me to go with Melanie to her home to check the situation there, which I did. Melanie and I went on the bus; she lived near a prison. Melanie and I worked through very paranoid and painful thoughts and feelings regarding her neighbours having gone into her flat with knives and trying to kill her many times. I heard her terror of felt or actual intrusions in her sense of being and considered how difficult this must have been for her alone in her flat.

When trying to enter her flat, we had to literally both push our bodies against the front door to this council flat due to walls of large laundry bags filled with clothes, books and many other objects that Melanie had wanted or needed to keep for any reasons. The several rooms were completely full of similarly loaded bags piled up halfway to the ceiling. I had never seen anything like it. Melanie said that she had been told that the flat would be deep cleaned. I was alert to discussing with Melanie any items that she wanted since the whole lot may disappear with the council deep clean. Melanie had clearly been hoarding, and she offered the insight, which was that she hoarded to block out the intruders. She and I started sifting through some of the bags, and many of the items were black magic rituals, which she discussed with me. I will never forget my fear sitting in her flat: the paranoia, her unpredictability, the sense of violence which I have never forgotten, the suffocating prison feel of her flat and the black magic perhaps irrationally made me feel vulnerable. Yet I was able to focus on the task at hand and on Melanie's needs as a traumatised and, therefore, very vulnerable young woman.

When we returned to the ward, Melanie and I had planned a therapy session. In this session, the neighbours came into her mind again as intrusive and dangerous, wanting to kill her. Melanie's mental state changed a great deal, which was bewildering to some extent. Her flat clearly and understandably stirred up a lot of anxiety for her, but I reflected to myself whether I was doing the therapy 'right'. I decided to follow Melanie and recognise what her state of mind was in any given moment. I decided to challenge her illusions and question what was happening for her. I asked if she thought that she was really being singled out by her neighbours, therefore, questioning her belief system. Melanie was able to think about reality and managed to do so in this session, perhaps a part of her that is non-psychotic. I wanted to help Melanie realise a part of her that can manage reality, a side of her that can be strengthened and brought out. It was in this session that Melanie decided she was going to work to afford to buy her daughter nice things.

It seems that there was a part of Melanie that felt utterly shattered and very deeply vulnerable but another part that survives, wants to work and works in the session. This session reminded me of Bion's reflections on the psychotic and non-psychotic parts of the personality (Bion, 1955). I wondered as I looked at her, 'What is there inside her?' perhaps a mix of rational and irrational thinking, waiting to see what comes on top. Part of her appeared omnipotent, a self-destructive self, reminding me of Rosenfeld's depiction of an internal mafia gang. Rosenfeld describes how he considers that narcissism represents the idealisation of the 'bad' parts of the self, felt as a gang, who can be turned to as a superior source of strength, becoming mobilised in a deliberate and organised attack on the dependent self and its rational object-relations (Rosenfeld, 1971). Perhaps there is a part of Melanie that she tries to keep on top of the paranoid, 'mad' and vulnerable side of herself.

It seemed that Melanie was presenting a dynamic/conflict that she is struggling with all of the time, supporting reality-based thinking.

Melanie makes reference to her dress in some therapy sessions, asking me if I like it. Melanie seems to be introducing in an indirect way the issue of not just what she looks like but what is she like inside, and again, this struggle is brought to me. Melanie was perhaps asking if she was black, evil or mad inside herself or smart or good at what she does. She didn't seem to know and looked in the mirror, seeming to doubt what she was like inside. In our exchange, I made reference to her internal world, where it was most significant for her, and she dealt with it concretely by evacuating her inside self; if I made reference to her internal world, she must have left a door open, like the neighbour who would persecute her, and unwillingly, I stirred up her feelings to evacuate them. Melanie had dealt with this in a less psychotic way; the door in her mind appeared to be left open, open for her to talk and see her internal state. She can then represent in her mind, through the neighbours, what is managed in the substitute representation. It seemed that there was a possibility of working at a more interpretative level. My clinical supervisor recognised this shift and indicated for me to try making occasional interpretations about her internal world, which would support the psychotic part of her.

The reality-based side of her, which wants to go to work, supports her ability to be rational, like in coming to see me. There appeared an incentive of her going to work in terms of her internal conflict. Going to work was perhaps a way of maximising the non-psychotic part of herself. Melanie had shared with me instances of when she had been socially inappropriate, such as not leaving a shop or blocking someone whom she found attractive from being able to go past. It seemed that the worry she has was of the psychotic part that can take over, which she wanted me to support her with. The psychotic, irrational side can become an encapsulated part of her, perhaps projecting her worry into me for me to put into words – her conflict, her worry. I tried to support the non-psychotic part of herself by intervening in her conflict to strengthen the stronger part of her.

I was well-trained in home visiting by that point and had thought through plans A and B etc., in case Melanie suddenly turned against me when just she and I alone in her flat. Additionally, I was aware of treading softly in her private living space and felt privileged to be invited into her fragile living environment, presumably imbued with experiences from family life over her lifetime. I hoped to establish in her mind a safer place for her to be, and I think that with careful thought, this was achieved to some extent. I am moved that Melanie shared a great deal with me on those home visits, and her fears of neighbours intruding lessened, as we examined the evidence for her fears. Melanie's main fears were neighbours intruding at night, but gradually, she was able to link the internal fears she understandably had with the external reality, which was that currently, there were no real threats. I suggested that she and I go and meet with the neighbours, which we planned to do, and over time, she told me that this was not necessary since her fears had subsided, which I was cautious about. She felt that she could move back to her flat and stay the night on her own. I supported her consistently in the transition from ward to home, and I was aware how difficult this experience can be for patients, especially those predominantly on their own. I am aware just how much patients with paranoid schizophrenia go through daily; we really need to understand better the needs of these individuals both on wards and in the community. I hope that I can convey some of what I have learned to be put into practice – realising the fragility and strengths of individuals who experience paranoia, taking them away from reality and offering boundaried, supportive attention to the detail of their needs. Careful listening and observation, I think, help a great deal, alongside consistency and reliability of relationship.

Melanie asked me if I would support her weekly once she was in the community. I wanted to support her therapeutically, and the ward consultant stated that this would be a private arrangement between Melanie and I, once she was established in the community. Clearly, my role was an adjustment that I needed to manage safely, in discussion with my clinical supervisor of 15 years, Professor Robert Hinshelwood. He was encouraging of me to continue my work with Melanie privately, and we discussed in detail how to set this up. Melanie started attending twice-weekly sessions, which went well, mainly due to my personal analysis, the extent of my direct experience of working with adults with a diagnosis of schizophrenia and the excellent supervision that I had also gained from psychiatrists, who were additionally trained psychoanalytically.

By 2012, four years into my therapy with Melanie, I had noticed that when I considered her thought disorder was improving – and, therefore, her perception of the world – her presentation would move back to one of psychosis, as demonstrated in this session:

### Thursday, 9 August 2012, 11:00

*Melanie is wearing a black wig, glasses and bright-red lipstick. For the first time that I have seen her in therapy, she is wearing a brightly coloured dress, showing her skin.*

HH: Hello, Melanie, do you want to come in?

M: (smiling) Yes, thanks.

HH: I notice that you are smiling today.

M: Yes, I feel happy; that is why. I have been to see my first child, Naomi. She is 5 years old now, she is lovely, and she is my daughter and always will be. They can't take away that from me. My mother can't take that away from me however hard she tries (looks glum).

HH: I see, so you have seen Naomi, which is a big thing for you. You look happy and then less happy when you are talking about your mother.

M: Yes, she makes me feel down about myself and seems always to be grabbing at what I have my photos of Naomi as if she is hers. I fear that what I have is going to be taken from me by her. It's a horrible feeling, as if I have to hold everything close and keep my eyes open when she is around. If I don't, something will be whipped away and then gone.

*HH:*   Perhaps you feel that you need to protect yourself from your mother?

*M:*    Yes, I do all of the time, all of the time, all of the time (becomes tearful).

*HH:*   It must be difficult for you, being a mother and these feelings coming up about your own mother.

*M:*    Yes, I can see now that it is bound to be, isn't it? That when I see my daughter, it brings up loads of pain about my own lack of a mother I feel.

*HH:*   Yes, that is very painful.

*M:*    And that I am not there for my daughter like my mother isn't there for me in the way that I need her to be. She intrudes on me and puts me down and won't listen to me as if I am a mad black bitch, who is not worth listening to or who has anything valuable to say (mumbles mad black bitch).

*HH:*   I value what you have to say here.

*M:*    Yes, I feel valued here. Perhaps I need you to give me what my mother cannot or will not give me. I feel that she will not give me what I need, then she is in a better place than me. She always said, 'Make sure that there is someone worse off than yourself', but I don't like that idea. I think that it is mean and violent. She is violent to me. I realise that now – that I have to swallow a lot of her violence – and I don't fight back.

*HH:*   What stops you from fighting back?

*M:*    I feel guilty that I was raped when I was 8 and that that has upset her and that that made daddy go away – that it is my fault. I feel that if I fight back, she will get hurt, that I will make her ill or that she will kill me or hurt me, so I keep my thoughts to myself.

*HH:*   Perhaps you would like to share some of those thoughts here with me.

*M:*    Yes, it's amazing, but I never thought that I would ever be in this situation when someone is saying what you are saying, to share my thoughts with them. I have been so alone for so long amongst my sisters and parents and never have I had the opportunity to share what I am feeling or thinking because I don't think it's worth tuppence, that I may hurt someone and so I store it all inside, like a rancid monster brewing away that I hope that no one will notice.

*HH:*   You hold onto your thoughts and feelings and don't let anyone in to be able to know them?

*M:*    No, I shouldn't let anyone in; otherwise, they may see who I am really and then something horrible would happen to me, worse than has happened already.

*HH:*   And who do you think that is?

*M:*    A horrible person (turns away).

*HH:*   Perhaps you are very sensitive about this, Melanie?

*M:*    (slowly turns back towards me and raises her eye to hold contact) I feel horrible inside. I feel that I am a monster and that I am horrible, but now, as I am sitting here, it doesn't seem so bad that you can see me and that you are not horrified. I thought that you would be horrified by seeing me. Why are you not (tearful and then angry)? Tell me why you are still looking at me and not repulsed by me. I have been hiding a part of me for years, ashamed of it, scared of being seen, frightened that I will be told to go to my room, locked up, sectioned, abandoned and left to die. I can't believe that you are still sitting with me normally. You don't look horrified or hurt or repulsed. I don't understand why not when I have thought all of my life that I am repulsive. I have wasted all of my life thinking that about myself, and now I let you see a bit of me, and nothing happens like I thought it would in my mind. I feel a huge loss, a huge loss of wasted life worrying about something that doesn't need to be worried about (sobs deeply for ten minutes or so).

*HH:*  I feel your sense of loss, too, Melanie.

*M:*  You have seen the most repulsive part of me, and you are still happy to talk to me. Why? I don't understand.

*HH:*  I feel privileged that you share your thoughts and feelings with me, Melanie. I think that you are realising that a part of you that you thought was repulsive actually isn't.

*M:*  Yes, I feel free of all of that worry. My mind is relaxing and clearing by the second (smiles broadly). There is no reason for me to have to hold all of that pain anymore. I can't believe it, how stupid I have been, people telling me bad things about myself and I believed it. What nasty shits (looks angry). How dare they talk to me like that (tearful)?

*HH:*  Yes, yes, it seems that you are facing something significant today about yourself and others.

*M:*  I feel relieved, and I feel that I have been stupid listening to all of those horrible things about myself, what nasty people.

*HH:*  Who are you talking about?

*M:*  My mother and one of my sisters. She is always putting me down like my mum, and they gang up on me.

*HH:*  Do you still think that you wouldn't stand up for yourself?

*M:*  No, I would stand up for myself. That is what I have not been doing and that's how they have managed to make me feel so bad. It's so obvious now.

*HH:*  Yes, when the veil lifts from the mind, often aspects of life seem so obvious, and I think you have faced something here today that will be life-changing for you.

*M:*  (face aglow) Yes, something big has changed today. I feel less vulnerable and stronger and able to see more clearly and to be able to say what is right and what is wrong.

*HH:*  A lot is changing then.

*M:*  Yes, I am amazed. It reminds me of the dream that I wrote down this morning (takes a paper from her pocket and reads). 'I was spreading green glitter paste all over my stomach with my right hand, there were other people around but not noticing me, I felt perturbed. I was in a house and a car came to pick me up, then went and I was still there and the car came again and picked someone else up. There was someone ill and I was asking that person all about their activity what they have been doing and what they are going to do, like they needed looking after'.

HH: It may be about the part of you that may need looking after at the moment.

M: I long for someone to look after me just sometimes (sobs suddenly and loudly).

HH: Yes, that's right. You are mourning the loss of having someone to hold the little girl.

M: (rocks gently) My little girl hurts and is confused. Why did that boy hurt me (sobs)? I didn't deserve that.

HH: No, you didn't deserve that.

M: No (cries).

HH: No, you didn't deserve that.

M: Poor me, poor little me. Sorry, sorry, it won't happen again.

HH: You perhaps feel compassion for yourself.

M: Yes, I had another dream that has just come back to me: *'I rang on this doorbell and a blonde girl opened the door a bit, looked at me and then closed it a bit and walked away leaving the door open saying sorry but walked back into this building. The girl was wearing a cream-coloured scarf and I saw her disappearing up the stairs. I went to the ledge which is outside on the street and looked through my bag. I went into this building and waited at the bottom of the stairs sitting in a chair feeling wretched. The therapist was a man and wouldn't let me see him because he had given my time to someone else. After I had waited wondering what they were doing, the therapist left saying that he couldn't see me because he was going out with the girl. I felt numb and left with them joining a crowd of people who seemed to be on a walking event. They were jolly and appreciated me being there'.*

HH: That's interesting. In your dream, you seem to have been excluded and afraid that you may be losing your place here and then part of a big friendly group of people.

M: Yes, I liked being part of the big group of people. They liked me, and I felt loved and happy.

HH: Perhaps you would like to belong to a group of friends, like in your dream, to feel liked and loved?

M: Yes, I would really like that (smiles broadly aglow).

HH: Well, let's think next Tuesday about different ways that you can make friends, people with similar interests.

M: Yay (childishly), I like that idea, something normal where I can belong.

HH: Yes, that is very important for everyone to have a sense of belonging.

M: Okay, I'll think about it.

HH:   Now, we need to stop for now.
M:     Okay, thanks very much. I feel much, much, much (childishly) better.
HH:   I'm glad you feel better, and see you on Tuesday.
M:     Okay, goodbye.

My work with Melanie required careful working through observation, reflection and supervision, alongside being gently supportive, increasing in frequency to four, sometimes five, times weekly, at her request. Melanie wanted to lie on the couch for comfort. Melanie and I discussed her want to lie on the couch, and considering that she would not see my face, I wondered how this would play out. I was cautious not to fuel possible obsessive-compulsive or addictive elements in Melanie and discussed these matters in depth with my supervisor, Professor Robert Hinshelwood. Over time, she managed to clear her flat and start to get to know her neighbours. Becoming Christian, Melanie gave up seeing and paying a spiritualist minister, which seemed to feed into her paranoia. Melanie started joining groups and tentatively established relationships through church, support groups and yoga and pilates. It took a lot of work over nine years for Melanie to be able to be in such groups due to her paranoia, anxiety and sense of agitation. Then Melanie started volunteering, then gaining paid employment as an assistant administrator. A turning point for Melanie was on visiting her father in Africa, as the following session shows:

### Tuesday, 24 October 2017, 8 AM

Session overview: *'Melanie'* – I have been seeing Melanie since 2008, mainly four and five times a week, with some breaks, for example, in 2016, when she travelled to Africa to stay with her father for six months. I have been working with her in a psychoanalytically informed supportive therapy; however, since returning from Africa, her more normal parts of her personality have shown themselves, and I have found that I can increasingly, though very cautiously, start to make occasional tentative psychoanalytic interpretations, which she can think about.

M:     Hi, Hi (wearing a black suit). I've changed my dress. Do you like it? Do you think that I look too black (lies on couch)? I am used to asking my sisters what they think, whether they think that I look okay because sometimes I can't see myself in the mirror. I looked in the mirror, and I couldn't tell whether I look okay or not.
T:     I think that you look smart.
        (pause)
        I wonder, Melanie, what stops you from being able to look in the mirror and see for yourself that you look *okay*.
M:     I don't know. I don't know. It's these drugs that I am on, I think. They make me feel hazy and lost. I am lost to my mummy and daddy. They left. They left me, and I didn't know where I was anymore. You hate me, I think.

T:    I am with you here, Melanie, and wonder if you feel distanced from me asking you about looking in the mirror that what I am saying may frighten you a little.

M:    (takes blanket and covers her body) I feel frightened, yes. Mummy and daddy left me.

T:    Perhaps you feel that I leave you by asking questions.

M:    I am trying to think. I am trying, but when I look in the mirror, I don't see me. It's all hazy and mucked up. What I see is a blur, and I can't see me. I'm a different person in the mirror than when I look at me not in the mirror.
(silence)

T:    I wonder if you and I can think about this because, apart from seeing yourself in the mirror, you can't see much of yourself otherwise. You can't see your own face apart from in the mirror.

M:    I catch myself in the window. I smile and catch myself and think, 'There you are. There you are. Don't worry. No worried Mel. You are there'. And I like it, but when I look in the mirror, I can't see. But sometimes I think that God lets me see myself, and I can kind of see myself. But from a distance, I'm out of myself and looking at myself, and I call that person looking at myself Zabia, Aunty Zabia looking at Mel, looking after little Mel. God helps me with this, I think. I think that God sends this angel to look after me, to comfort me and to help me, like a parent but an aunt, a female.

T:    Hmm, I am interested in what you are saying and wonder if, as you and I have talked about previously, whether you not getting on so well with your mother creates this need for an aunt-type figure, who looks after you but that that person is inside of you, from your need for a mother.

M:    She looks like you (laughs loudly and manically for a long time, then cries, farts loudly and laughs again). I need to go to the toilet. I need to go. Sorry. Sorry, I be back.
(Melanie returns from the toilet after five or so minutes.)
Clean now. Had to let it all out. Sorry. I am back (lies on couch), naughty Melanie like a baby.

T:    Yes, you are back now. Hmmm, I am interested, Melanie, in what you are saying. You are saying that the part of you that looks at you looks like me.

M:    Yes, but I mean that I quite like that I don't run away and hide like I did with my mummy and daddy when they argued and fought when I was younger. I can stay a bit more like me when I see you watching over me, like you do here, I suppose. But when I am not here, it happens, not when I am here.

T:    I see that you can sometimes sense my presence when you are not here. I appear, or your aunt appears, who looks like me, and you can stay you when your aunt, who looks like me, is there.

M:    Yes, like here, I can stay me more and for longer, rather than feel that I need to run away and hide, but there is nowhere to run and hide to because it is me. I can't run out of my body. I just want to disappear sometimes when I see my mummy in my mind. I want to close my eyes and die and run away, but I can't run from myself, or I would die. I have wanted to die before because I can't run out of my body. I have to stay with my body, but the only way out is to die. It's sad (cries). Poor Melanie, baby girl. Melanie, baby girl (rocks with arms). Melanie needs mummy. The baby needs mummy love.

T:    Perhaps you are saying that you have found a way to comfort the baby part of yourself.

M:    I need to. I need to. I look in the mirror, and my mind escapes from the mirror. I am frightened by it. I can't see myself there, but I can here and when my aunt appears. I have wanted to die, and once, my neighbours were going to do it for me. They came into my flat with knives and were going to kill me, and I was afraid. I phoned the police and told them calmly what was happening, and when they arrived, they found my door wide open and asked me why I was leaving my door open. And I said that I was letting my neighbours in because they wanted to kill me with knives.

T:    Melanie, but maybe you are saying that you wanted them to kill you.

M:    Yes, it was go telling them and me that my time had come and that I wanted to die and they wanted me to die and God did, too, so that was agreed. I was going to die, and I had to leave the door open to let that happen.

T:    And you are telling me this now alive and just having been promoted.

M:    Yes, for some reason, God must have been called to do something else because I am alive. I know that I realise that I am alive now talking to you, but it must have been because at that time, about five years ago, God was called to another job to do more important because he has so much in the world to do, but he is often looking out for me, too, telling me what to do, what to eat and not eat. I don't eat anything from super-markets because God has told me that poison is in the food sent by the Russians. I eat food from smaller shops not connected with Russians.

T:    You believe that the food in supermarkets is contaminated by Russians, but why would people spend time doing that, Melanie?

M:    I don't know. I don't know, but I know that God has warned me about it, and I listen to him. I listen, you know. God is good so that is why. You don't understand (looks back at me fiercely)?

T:    I eat from supermarkets, and I am here talking with you, and I enjoy the food I cook from supermarkets.

M:    (turns fiercely) You say that you say that (sulks).

T:    I am interested that you perhaps don't like me contradicting what you believe, Melanie.

*M:*   (silence, cross looking) I am thinking about what you said, and I don't like it because how is it that you can eat food from supermarkets and be alive when I can't? Why is it that I am singled out by the Russians to make the food bad for me when you eat from supermarkets? I don't understand it, although I can see that it can't be true, can it? I can't be the only one who is singled out because they wouldn't be able to tell which food I was going to buy so that can't be true. I feel stupid, and I feel angry that I am being told lies, that who has led me to believe that I can't eat food from supermarkets. It's stupid, and I seem to fall for this crap all of the time. I'm not going to continue living out someone else's lie for them.

*T:*   I wonder, Melanie, if those aspects that you think are outside of you may be inside you that you and I could start to think about together. We can talk about it together if you want to.

*M:*   Yes, God is there, but you seem to say that God is in me too (smiles). Thank you. Thank you. That is lovely to hear, so lovely, I feel really good, really agreeable with you. God is in me.
(silence)
That's good. God smiles on me. God is light.

*T:*   I am curious about how you feel now about going into supermarkets.

*M:*   Hmm, mixed, I guess. I guess about how I feel because it's hard to say, all sorts of different characters mixed up. How does anyone of them feel at any one time? it's hard, but I am thinking about what you are saying because you are alive and eat from supermarkets and so the food can't be poisoned (turns around and looks at me pleadingly and puzzled). It's a strange one for me because God is involved, I thought. I thought God was involved.
(silence)
I don't quite get it, but I trust you. God has been telling me only to eat fruit and nuts because they were there in the Garden of Eden, where shame was discovered. I have had to eat fruit and nuts because the Bible only mentions fruit but then you said nuts were there, too, so I ate nuts, too, and found that they are good for me. Fruit and nuts are good for me.

*T:*   Perhaps you can think of other foods that were there.

*M:*   (long silence) I think that there were animals too. I think but not fish.

*T:*   There was no water, but Noah lived on a ship.

*M:*   (long silence) Yes, that's true. There would have been fish and birds and animals to eat.

*T:*   I realise that we need to stop for now, but let's meet tomorrow at 8 AM.

*M:*   (puzzled looking) Yes, there were birds there and fishes. I'm okay for work today. Thank you. Bye, bye.

It meant a great deal to Melanie to have seen her father, and from then, she was promoted to a managerial role. She also met someone to whom she felt romantically inclined towards and was able to sustain this relationship, which positively changed her.

In supervised therapy with me, Melanie grew able to think more about herself and others, but I realistically always held in mind an underpinning fragility that needed to be held in mind and treated with great caution and care.

By 2018, I was able to work psychoanalytically with Melanie, as the following session may illustrate.

### Tuesday, 15 May 2018, 7 AM

*M:*    It's . . . it's . . . it's upsetting. I think that sometimes the sun is talking to me, or being warm just for me, warming my spirit so that I can live, be alive. And it warms me to know that the sun is my friend but more than that, like a mother to me, keeping me alive, those warm warming tones of speaking to me, yellow swirls, moving to white in the centre, my love.

*T:*    The sun is like a mother to you.

*M:*    Kind of like that, mother sun, mother sun. I had a dream last night. It was a dream. It was a dream that left me feeling scared. I was in a corridor and walked round, and there was a room with people in it. And one lady walked out of the room to meet me in the corridor, and I held her by the shirt and twisted it and said, 'I will kill you if you speak about me again'. It was someone that I used to work with in the past, but the person who I said this to wasn't someone that I had disliked. It was someone who I was competitive with, though, in the past at work. I think because the boss can only promote certain people.

*T:*    It's an interesting dream. I want to go back if that is okay to ask you if the person who you spoke to is like anyone.

*M:*    She's like my second eldest sister, 'B', who I have felt competitive with all of my life. She's been good to me, and I love her, but sometimes she can be a pig. She is like a dirty whore sometimes because of the things that she says to me. She calls me a dirty whore when I was a child, like my dad called my mum sometimes, and I hated her for that. 'B' was kind to me, too, though, but I remember once when I was little that she asked me to pee through a tube, and of course, I couldn't do it. I felt ashamed by that. I hated myself for not having been able to do it, then to have done it knowing that I couldn't do it but that she had shamed me like that. I started hitting myself after that, slapping myself around the face when I was in a room on my own, or I would just slap myself without being in control of what I was doing. Where was my mummy and daddy then? Why didn't they look after me then? It was very terrible for me – that event.

*T:*    It's a difficult memory for you.

M:    Yes, although really, I should be able to get over it, and actually hearing myself telling you, it isn't so bad actually. Really, it was perhaps worse than it was. I see little dark figures running around when I think about this. I see strange little dark figures altogether running around in a row for some reason when I think of this memory. Why is that (turns to look at me)?
(silence)
M lies back down.

T:    Perhaps you need to check me.

M:    I did. I needed to see that you weren't one of the little black figures, which doesn't make sense because they are males and you are clearly female. It's weird in one way because I have known you for a long time, and I trust you, but still, you can change in my mind like that from someone that I trust to someone that is male and a little dark figure (laughs). Melanie, you are a very silly girl. What are you talking about, silly Melanie, silly girl? You are a crazy pup.

T:    You speak in a different voice, and I wonder if those words have been said to you before.

M:    Oh! You mean what I have just said? Yes, that is me when I was a girl and how my sister used to speak to me. She thought that I was crazy and said that I did weird things, like eat jam on its own and wear my slippers to the park, things like that. But all of that seems fine to me. But she and my other sisters used to laugh, and I used to laugh with that at me as if I was separate that I was amongst the sisters laughing at me as if I was not separate.

T:    Yes, perhaps a part of you was laughing with your sisters at another part of you.

M:    Well, I think that it is okay to eat jam on its own. It's delicious and sweet, but I can also see the funny side of it because it's indulgent, and others don't eat jam on its own like me, well, not in public. But that doesn't mean that what I am doing is wrong because others don't do it. And going to the park in my slippers, well, it's comfy to do that. They are like shoes, and now it's the fashion. Shops are making a fortune out of people wearing slippers like they are day-to-day shoes. How long was that for the fashion industry to copy my idea (laughs for a long time)? Silly Melanie (laughs and then rocks herself, arms folded).
(long silence)
My dream is about my murderer inside me.
(long silence)
I can't tell anyone that. I hope that this is confidential, or I will be sectioned again. You wouldn't do that, would you, not to me, little Melanie, your little girl on the couch?
(pause)

T:    You fear me thinking about your dream in a way that may turn against you.

M:      Yes, no, yes (laughs). Does that answer your question? It's those dark men figures, the little men that I fear. They are in my head, and I fear that you are going to turn into one of them. I checked, and you are not, but I have to check. I have murderous feelings and that doesn't seem to be socially acceptable. People don't go round talking about their murderous feelings, but I can tell that others have them, like my sister, because I have such beautiful black hair and large brown eyes. She used to try and poke my eyes out and pull my hair. She even cut it in the night once. And I had to go to school wearing a hat, and my mummy gave me a wig, which didn't fit. And all the school laughed at me. It doesn't seem so bad telling you about that, but it was horrible at the time because underneath that awful wig that mummy gave me, I think that it was one of hers, was my hair all cut jagged by 'S' in the night. She hated my hair being so beautiful. She kept the cuttings in a scrapbook for years and years. She probably still has them. Who is crazier, though? My pain goes deep.

T:      You sound aware of your pain, and perhaps it feels okay to talk about it.

M:      Yes, I had a huge argument with mummy at the weekend because I don't see why I should take her talking about me in a bad way. I don't think that I am bad. You don't seem to think so, and my work doesn't seem to think so. And I don't think that I am bad either. I think that I have bad thoughts about knives and black magic and that I get very, very afraid and have frightening thoughts and they get darker and blacker and deeper and more and more away from the sun's rays of warm light, more like into a deep, dark hell, where the cauldron is brewing with different dark thoughts, full of malice and hurt.

        I feel lighter having had the argument with mummy because I don't cave in as I usually do. I usually feel like I am 4 or 5 or 7 or 8 and become childlike to her as I have always done, but this time, I stayed adult, stayed Melanie, and it felt good. I felt strong. I don't deserve to be treated badly by her. I feel that she is really nasty to me, like she isn't behaving like a mother, and she encourages my sisters to be nasty to me too. It's not like a loving mother no wonder I have suffered. But I stood strong, and she backed off and looked afraid. She is now the afraid one because she can't bully me no more (laughs). Good Melanie with the sun in her hair, good Melanie with the warm sun shining on me a smiling face, not one tortured by cruelty.

T:      You seem to be speaking of feeling stronger.

M:      (laughs) Isn't that the best news that you have heard recently? I am so, so happy. I never thought that I could stand strong like that and see my mum cower away. I was not cruel to her, or I did not say a nasty thought either, just stood strong. It was so effective, and I have never done that before. I have always felt that my mind is going to cave and collapse.

T:      You are pleased with yourself and perhaps proud.

*M:*    Yes, although I also have darker thoughts with the little black men who walk in a row, and I have to check who you are. Are you going to hurt me? Are you going to make me sad and like a child?

*T:*    Perhaps you being like a child is to be sad.

*M:*    Yes, of course. You know that, don't you by now? That my child is a sad one, that I was hated and hurt and that I see that my mummy was very, very cruel to me and that now I have grown up, she can't do it to me. It's because you have been kind to me and the people at work give me love and value that I have changed, I think, and it has shocked the wit out of my black mother, the black woman hell of my life.

*T:*    I see that we are coming to an end for today, but I wonder if you are going to work today.

*M:*    Yes, I am going to start on a new project that they have given me to set up a database using Edexcel and so I can learn a new programme and will be working with 'C', who I like.

*T:*    I will see you tomorrow.

*M:*    Bye.


**Reflections on my work with Melanie**

Melanie was clearly a psychotic patient with a lot of resources, to have managed the demands of gaining a degree, with the ongoing support of her sisters. My sense is of Melanie's psychological development was severely interfered with around the age of 8, when her father left and the rape occurred in the park, both abandoning experiences that likely left her too exposed and vulnerable, especially with an abusive mother. I was cautious to work with Melanie therapeutically on a permanent basis but continue to work with her today 15 years on with a supportive psychoanalytic frame, as encouraged by Professor Robert Hinshelwood, to persist with an analytic approach. The ethnic differences between Melanie and me were sensitively approached, to the extent that, from the start, a positive rapport was quickly established between Melanie and me on the ward, and trust was kindled through her pregnancy and birth, continuing through to the transition into the community, other relationships, work and romance.

I sensitively challenged Melanie's utterances that black people project their difficulties into their skin, suggesting that white people are historically more likely to do so. I further consistently challenged Melanie's sense that black people are not worth much and explored her thoughts and feelings about this, which was very painful. I was very careful in relation to Melanie's paranoid aspect of her personality, which perhaps could break out through her fragile psychic skin (Bick), and sensitivity was required to keep this in balance; I saw the good in her and communicated this with her. Malanie was not used to positive feedback, touching on inner pain in her, which I helped her with, and this seemed to create space to have more fruitful relationships. However,

I reflected on how compliments might seem like a form of saving her, for which she could feel gratitude, but could also switch to the opposite, and perhaps the more she switches, the more she may feel paranoid. Her ongoing reference to her lost babies sadly led me to wonder whether she felt full of corpses that needed to be mourned, reflecting how terrible she feels inside. Perhaps she is trying to keep her baby self alive by having more and more babies in a compulsive or delusional way, destroying life to start creating it again. I was often aware of being careful of not offering too much intimacy, since I felt that if this was felt to be too much for Melanie, she may want to smash it all. I wondered whether this was why she doesn't have friends, a sense that anyone can and did walk in and out of her life. I hoped that therapy could offer a mirror for her, as Winnicott describes – a mirror like that of the mother, a specific form of mirroring in therapy, reflecting her fragility and moments when she feels intruded upon by me. It seems that in therapy with individuals who tend towards psychosis, they are very sensitive to how genuine I am or whether I am trying to manipulate them. Over the course of the therapy, I wondered how much she can trust me and reflected deeply on how this affects her life.

It seemed that Melanie was able to recognise different realities through the course of the therapy, which is usually broken down in schizophrenia. Melanie appeared to be an isolated, autistic woman but was able to manage a wider spectrum of relationships through the course of therapy. At the start, however, she had wanted to talk with me, showing her propensity to sociability. Her relationship with her father appeared distant and idealised. I am unclear if Melanie would ever recover from her father having left her with her mother, who was not protective towards Melanie but, on the contrary, very destructive of her as a person, from my observations in person and from Melanie's accounts, listening closely to what was in her mind. I could respond to Melanie and recognise that her state of mind had changed and modify my interventions accordingly. I observed mainly two states of mind during the course of therapy, where Melanie described feeling 'horrible' or 'happy'. I considered these two parts of herself as unintegrated at the start of therapy but more so towards the present day, perhaps through assisting her to grieve and Melanie being more able to think about herself and, therefore, distinguish herself from her environment, including others' minds.

When Melanie spoke to me: 'I was talking to myself as if there were two of me, the listener and the speaker', this seemed to illuminate a problem of not knowing who she is and a task of integrating these parts of herself, bringing these parts together. Melanie shared about the listener part listening to the hallucinated voice, alongside her being the voice but in this state of hallucination, understandably not knowing quite who she is. These are separate and different aspects between speaker and listener, perhaps coming apart at the seams. In psychoanalytic terms, one would talk about the problem of the different parts, as outlined earlier. Mostly, Melanie's intent in her dreams was contained but not manifestly psychotic. She appeared through her dreams, at peace with herself later in the therapy, but this could quickly change to a paranoid-schizoid state versus an idealisation, which spoke of the awfulness of her state of mind. However, Melanie's projective evacuative quality of communication at times perhaps indicated eliminating what was desperate and intolerable, like a lavatory into me. Perhaps she becomes reacquainted with some of the horrible experiences in her life. Then things take over, and everything is either wonderful or everything is horrible quite unrealistically. And she veers between these states, as part of her psychotic process.

Melanie has demonstrated her inner resources, now in a senior managerial role (starting from a temporary administrative position) in 2012. Melanie has a partner of ten years with whom she now lives in a different flat from the one described earlier. She appears happy yet still struggles with paranoia, which she seems to manage through hoarding; the obsessive-compulsive component of her personality. Melanie has a group of friends whom she thinks she can rely on and has reestablished her relationships with her sister, with more stable boundaries with her mother and better communication with her father, whom she has visited five times during the course of the therapy. To her delight, Melanie managed to gain a master's degree in business administration and is setting up her own business. With more money, she is proud to be able to support her 15-year-old daughter more now, with whom she has a positive relationship and has been on holiday unsupervised several times. Their contact now is entrusted to Melanie, without social services intervention, unless she needs them. She wants to continue seeing me for a while longer to explore her early childhood more and to think about getting married to her partner.

# 11 Case study 7 – 'Aasiya'

'Nor aught so good but strained from that fair use,
Revolts from true birth stumbling on abuse'.

*Romeo and Juliet* – William Shakespeare

## Introduction

The following case study describes my systemic work with Family 'A' and a particular individual work with 'Aasiya'. This family (parents and ancestry) was born in India, but Aasiya and her siblings (Amar – sister; Ahmed and Kanesh – brothers) were born in the UK; the females wore hijabs, and all were practising Muslims. The family will be described using systemic concepts and theories, alongside the therapeutic system, approach and interventions used. Reference will be made to my self-reflexive practice and to relevant systemic literature. This case study will include information in terms of the following: the background to the referral, a systemic account of the family, an account of the course of therapeutic work and the relationship between the therapist and the family, ending and outcomes and my reflections and learning points. Let's now turn to consider the background to the referral.

## The background to the referral

'Family A' was referred to me for fortnightly, two-hourly, home-based family work in March 2018 via my website, the consultant psychiatrist requesting fortnightly feedback.

In the first home-based family meeting, I observed that 'Aasiya', the referred person, aged 45, appeared dependent on the NHS for safety; her family was hostile to the NHS, reminding me of the difficulties in relation to the treatment in terms of the referring person or organisation (Selvini-Palazzoli et al., 1980, p. 3. 'Aasiya' had been re-sectioned onto an inpatient psychiatric assessment ward due to suicidal and psychotic presentation. I worked on the ward with 'Aasiya' as an interpersonal psychotherapist, alongside the nursing team and medical staff. Aasiya confided in me within the bounds

DOI: 10.4324/9781003509059-12

of a developing professional, co-constructive relationship; allegedly, she had been sexually abused by her uncle 'Firoh' from the ages of 3–12 years old. Her father, 'Edhas', was reportedly also sexually abused, until the age of 13, by 'Firoh'. When 'Aasiya' managed to share with me about the sexual abuse, I felt deeply angry and saddened, reflecting on how this created an alliance in me with her, alongside negotiating professional distance. I recognised 'Aasiya's' varied needs on the ward, including her dependence on me for safety. I reflected on the impact of the transition in my role to that of family practitioner and her attachment style, which led to her understandably not wanting me out of her sight since, when she had been left on her own as a child, she had reportedly been abused. I considered the constraints of working safely in 'Aasiya's' home, revisiting guidelines from social work training.

At the referral meeting in March 2018, the psychiatrist's overriding concern was 'Aasiya's' extreme vulnerability, which I agreed with; she recommended family work as a supervisory intervention. 'Aasiya's' mental health observably deteriorated following a visit from her mother, 'Sanya', aged 70, and the high level of expressed emotion from 'Edhas' (her father), demonstrating severe volatility (Kuipers, 2006, p. 73). 'Aasiya's' narrative expressed her deep insecurity within the family, which was very painful to be aware of, especially in terms of the power dynamics; when discharged, she required 24-hour supervision due to suicidality risk. My initial hypothesis was that 'Aasiya' felt isolated, dependent and powerless in her family and needed to externalise the problems to explore her strengths rather than her vulnerabilities (White & Epston, 1990). The preferred outcome was regaining her position as mother to 'Kahini' (daughter) and 'Rakesh' (son) and feeling empowered in her family. I reflected on the similarities and differences between 'Family A' and my own, acknowledging my frustrations towards 'Edhas' and 'Sanya' (Aasiya's father and mother), mildly resonating with the issues of communication and responsibility in my family.

I reflected upon the different cultural positions of the NHS psychiatric services and the family system: 'Aasiya' depending on it for safety, 'Edhas' threatening 'Aasiya' with being sectioned to manage her understandably anxious, obsessive and dependent behaviours and 'Sanya' viewing Aasiya's time in hospital as respite, creating competition for caring (Selvini-Palazzoli et al., 1980, pp. 3–4). Sanya was harsh and cruel towards Aasiya in the visits to her on the ward, which was sad to witness and inevitably had a further negative impact on Aasiya. Perhaps Sanya's attitude towards Aasiya was to keep her in hospital.

We will now turn to consider the systemic account of the family.

## A systemic account of 'Family A'

'Family A' is structurally matriarchal, with 'Sanya', aged 70, 'Aasiya', aged 45, 'Kahini', aged 9, and Rakesh, aged 7, spanning three generations, living together as a mutual support system. I observed 'Sanya' making all decisions for 'Aasiya', despite Aasiya being very intelligent, presenting in the family script in the role of a symptomatic, vulnerable 'child', with 'Kahini' as a parental-child. The family structure is disorganised, a possible coalition appearing between 'Sanya', 'Kahini' and Rakesh to take charge of 'Aasiya' (Minuchin et al., 1978, pp. 20–21). 'Sanya' is separated from 'Edhas', aged 72, both parents to 'Aasiya', 'Amar', aged 38 (Aasiya's sister), 'Ahmed', aged 30, and Rakesh, aged 28. Three years ago, 'Edhas' met 'Ariti', aged 35, through networking, now father to a 2-year-old daughter, 'Bella'. The disorganised family structure is maintained by 'Sanya' accommodating the maternal role, which 'Aasiya' presents as not fulfilling, perhaps due to her chronic psychosis, suicidality and history of eating disorders, linked to medication stimulating weight-gain and weight-loss issues. In addition, there are child safeguarding issues regarding Kahini and Rakesh, putting me in an additional role in the realm of the domain of production (Lang et al., 1990).

In relation to the life-cycle transitions, 'Sanya' raised the question of who is going to look after 'Aasiya' when they die. Coordinated management of meaning (CMM) teaches the deontic logical interpretive questions of 'What are they doing?' and 'Why are they doing that?' to further think about what is said and unsaid in relation to who would meet 'Sanya's' needs if 'Aasiya' got better (Pearce, 2005, p. 39). A further transition involves 'Kahini' approaching pre-adolescence and Rakesh being in latency, leaving 'Aasiya' grieving for the loss of 'Kahini' and Rakesh in relation to her maternal role. As 'Kahini's' sexuality comes to the fore in adolescence, this possibly raises issues for 'Aasiya' regarding sexuality and being single, heightened by Aasiya's alleged experiences of abuse. 'Ali', aged 42, 'Kahini' and 'Rakesh's' father and 'Aasiya's' ex-husband, seeks contact with 'Aasiya', 'Kahini' and 'Rakesh'; contact was allowed by 'Sanya' only by letter due to his forensic history. Ali is serving a life sentence in prison for manslaughter, armed burglary and sexual assaults on women. Aasiya is understandably very fearful and distressed about when he may be released from prison and is extremely vulnerable to being persuaded to contact him, without properly being able to think through the consequences, due to her psychosis and need for attention and love. Additionally, 'Edhas' has a new partner, 'Ariti', and their daughter, 'Bella'.

A dominant narrative in the family relates to power differentials, namely, 'Aasiya' being unprotected as a child, 'Edhas' being aware of Firoh's alleged pedophilia and 'Sanya's' claims of being unaware of her daughter being abused for nine years. 'Aasiya' believes that her psychosis is caused by the sexual abuse; other family members not only disagree but they also dismiss the abuse. 'Aasiya' had allegedly been threatened by 'Firoh', such that if she told anyone about the abuse, he would do the same to 'Amar', 'Ahmed' and 'Kanesh'. 'Amar', 'Ahmed' and 'Kanesh', now successful professionals, breed resentment in relation to Aasiya. In contrast, 'Aasiya's' diminished functioning creates tensions, and I reflected on the CMM approach regarding 'multiple levels of embedded contexts' to understand multiple perspectives (Pearce, 2005, pp. 39–40). Additionally, a double-bind is created for 'Aasiya'. 'Edhas' believes that 'Aasiya' can do more. 'Sanya' believes that 'Aasiya' cannot be unsupervised, with or without 'Kahini' and 'Rakesh'.

Individual issues and risk are of child safeguarding in relation to 'Kahini', 'Ahmed' and 'Kanesh' and adult safeguarding in relation to 'Aasiya'. 'Aasiya' remains a high suicide risk. A further risk involves 'Ali's' contact with 'Sanya', who colludes with his wishes, at the cost of 'Aasiya's' sense of safety and psychological stability, who is terrified of 'Ali'.

The context is one of a wealthy, middle-class Asian family, who had provided a seemingly financially privileged upbringing to their daughters and sons in the UK. 'Aasiya's' breakdown at 19 years old, preceded her later disclosure to 'Edhas' about the abuse. 'Edhas' then disclosed to 'Aasiya' about his. It is medically documented that 'Aasiya' had been hospitalised with Anorexia Nervosa at age 8 years old, her parents denying this, raising concerns for me about her well-being in the present. Since aged 19, 'Aasiya' has had many psychiatric hospital admissions due to not taking her medication and suffering subsequent psychotic breakdowns.

At the age 22, 'Aasiya' attended university to study medical anthropology, meeting 'Ali', whom she married at age 28, then parenting 'Kahini' and 'Rakesh', with 'Sanya' as the main consistent parent. In terms of issues of power and difference, 'Sanya' has a dominant script. 'Edhas's' volatile behaviour is being dismissed, perhaps through a cross-generational coalition. 'Kahini' and 'Rakesh' support 'Sanya' with this but, at the same time, are resentful for their mother's incapacity. Although 'Aasiya' conveys powerlessness, her illness controls the whole family, with reciprocal controlling of 'Aasiya' by 'Sanya' and possibly 'Ali'. 'Aasiya' seems to hold the role of the vulnerable child in the family, expressed through her seeming irresponsibility.

In relation to social constructionism, 'Family A's' narrative is based on 'Aasiya's' suicidality and psychosis, which organises the whole family. 'Sanya' believes that 'Aasiya' is unable to do daily tasks, perhaps maintaining control of 'Aasiya'. 'Aasiya's' beliefs are of anticipated harm to herself and her family, and her regrets about the past for which she feels responsible, perhaps revealing her unfinished grieving process.

A genogram tracks the historical and current patterns of relationship (McGoldrick et al., 2008). I completed a genogram with the family, which, as predicted, caused a great deal of argument, which was managed sensitively and firmly in a later session of family work.

We will now turn to my account of the therapeutic work and the relationship between 'Family A' and myself.

### An account of the course of therapeutic work and the relationship between the therapist and the family

The aim of this section is to show my thinking about the process of family therapy to examine the relationship between therapist and family and the decisions about interventions and the family's response to those interventions. The model(s) of therapy used will be described briefly and illustrated within this section. An account of the involvement or influence of the wider therapeutic team will also be outlined.

My experience of the referral process from the NHS was positive due to the psychiatrist adopting a low-key position. Home-based family work commenced in March 2013, with all adults attending most of the 23 sessions to date. 'Kahini', 'Rakesh', 'Ahmed' and 'Kanesh' did not want to attend the sessions, and I was curious as to why not.

The early phase of therapy involved co-constructing the boundaries and limits, according to the Association of Family Therapy (AFT); it appeared easy to join and engage the family's trust. The aims of the therapy were discussed, 'Aasiya's' situation being the focus. I reflected on my values as a therapist being curious, fair, boundaried, respectful, humble and a spontaneous agent for change in terms of the interplay of person and context. The family's presence, my observations and my participation in their verbal and non-verbal communications conveyed a willingness to let me into their system. However, I re-clarified the limits of my role, in the light of attempts to render me inoperative, by trying to absorb me into the family and continuously inviting me for meals. I was informed by the 'stickiness' of blurred boundaries in the family. My approach was one of 'permission-seeking' (Aggett et al., 2011), for example, asking, 'Is it okay to come in?' and 'Would it be alright to sit in this chair?' to empower them. Whilst 'Aasiya' responded well to permission-seeking, 'Edhas' and 'Sanya' considered it manipulative, lending weight to my initial hypothesis about 'Aasiya's' disempowerment and her parents blocking my empowerment of her.

I used circular questioning to further test my hypothesis and include all family members in the position of observers to themselves to introduce 'not too unusual difference' and change (Andersen, 1990). This intervention brought feelings and thoughts alive in the family, which I listened to closely, asked further questions about and resumed active listening. I attended to my own feelings of comfort/discomfort and those of the family to maintain safety of the session for improvisation (Byng-Hall, 1995). With the essential Milan principles held in mind of 'Hypothesizing-Circularity-Neutrality' (Selvini-Palazzoli et al., 1980), the main issues arising in the first two sessions were 'Aasiya's' sense of powerlessness, housing situation and relationship with 'Kahini' and 'Rakesh' (grandchildren) and respite for 'Sanya'. A second hypothesis was this: If 'Aasiya' wasn't psychotic, how different would life be? This was formulated with the intention of generating ideas about the nature of what was going on in the family, 'stimulating the family to produce meaningful information' (Selvini-Palazzoli et al., 1980, p. 1). I asked 'Edhas' the miracle question in the first session (Berg & Nolan, 2001, p. 7), and his answer and other members' responses established the basis for future sessions.

Power and difference emerged as an issue early on, noticing conflict between 'Edhas's' precarious role in the family and mine, perhaps indicating vulnerability. To address this, I asked 'Edhas' the future-oriented question: If 'Aasiya' was not psychotic, what are the taboos that would come up? 'Edhas' was able to express his fears intelligently as a result. However, I reflected that 'Edhas' expected more radical changes than I offered, with 'Aasiya' being given daily tasks to do. His response communicated frustration about 'Aasiya', yet it then emerged that 'Edhas' considers that he suffers from milder symptoms than those of 'Aasiya'.

Early on, a conversation unfolded regarding denial by 'Sanya' and 'Edhas' of 'Aasiya' having suffered from Anorexia Nervosa, despite documentation in the medical records. 'Amar' and 'Kanesh' endorsed awareness of Aasiya's diagnosis of Anorexia Nervosa, a coalition emerging between 'Aasiya' and 'Amar' (sister), with 'Edhas' as the third in the triad in disaccord. 'Sanya's' and 'Edhas's' denial of historical facts conveyed patterns of distortions in communication, indicating difficulties of differences in the family and the double-bind for 'Aasiya', where her parents invalidated her reality in the context of psychosis. It appeared impossible for me to remain neutral at the same time considering whether I was being drawn into an unethical situation, feeling allied with 'Aasiya', 'Amar' and 'Kanesh', perhaps due to being closer to their age and having a sense of truth. I considered that I was, perhaps, tainted by my prejudices in relation to my feelings of anger towards 'Sanya' and 'Edhas' about 'Aasiya's' childhood and in the present in relation to 'Sanya's' contact with 'Ali', despite 'Aasiya's' distress and severe paranoia made worse by this contact. I hypothesised that 'Edhas' and 'Sanya' perhaps didn't want the victim ('Aasiya') removed from this role. I wondered about the function this role performed for them. Perhaps if Aasiya is psychotic, her narrative of sexual abuse can be dismissed, relieving them of their responsibilities as parents.

From session four, it seemed important to establish a shared sense of reality in the family. 'Aasiya' asked her parents what they thought she was in hospital for when she was 8 years old, leading to their acknowledgement of her suffering and their absence of care. This led to exploring the different relational needs in the family and reflecting back to the family using empowering sentences, such as 'What you are teaching me is . . . ' or 'You've taught me that . . . '. It was essential to attempt to free myself from the 'linguistic and cultural conditioning', for example, 'Sanya' instructing me: 'You agree, don't you?' I attempted tracking family beliefs from session five onwards. I questioned my own prejudices and beliefs, especially my assumption that reality exists, considering Cecchin's words that 'It is a prejudice to say that reality exists . . . what we see, we are creating it'.

The conflict in my responsibility as a family therapist, between the domains of exploration and social control and assessing safeguarding in the domain of production, was a prevalent issue in relation to 'Aasiya', 'Kahini', 'Rakesh' and 'Bella' and a struggle in terms of maintaining my stance of curiosity (Cecchin, 1987, p. 3). Being the sole therapist highlighted the importance of talking with my mentors in order to remain curious.

In the fifth session, a main circular pattern of behaviour observed was the dominance of 'Edhas' in relation to the predominantly female membership of the family. A challenge was remaining curious in relation to 'Edhas' due to his, at times, dismissiveness of his family's and my views. I was helped by experienced practice that 'therapeutic responsibility begins with seeing your own position in the system' and my lack of power (Cecchin, 1987, p. 3).

The following interaction illustrates the reframing of a typical circular pattern of behaviour by posing a future-oriented circularity:

*'Edhas':*    Why are you defending him? He's a murderer. Good choice, 'Sanya', well done.

*Therapist:* Perhaps 'Sanya' defending 'Ali' suggests that she feels threatened and trapped in the family. I'm wondering how you want things to be different.

*'Aasiya':*   I don't feel that I have a place in the family, but I love them very much. They are everything to me.

By reframing, followed by connotation, I hoped to give 'Aasiya's' behaviour meaning in connection to the family system and to positively connote the intention behind her behaviour. My aim was to separate 'Aasiya's' behaviour from her person and to acknowledge and regulate the double-binds and paradoxes that emerged through the communication patterns. On reflection, I would be cautious about using paradox in the future.

I considered that I was posing understanding to prescribe a change in behaviour connected to the rules of family therapy as opposed to the rules in the family system, presenting as intolerance of difference in their children. The difference in the rules was reflected on by 'Edhas', offering direction for change, but I wondered whether he behaved differently outside family work. Aasiya reported Edhas easily losing his temper and regularly shouting at her. She felt sympathy towards him for having gone through sexual abuses like her and perhaps endured this hurtful attitude towards her.

I wondered how my gender, age and race impacted my relationship with 'Family A' (Zimmerman, 2001, p. 34) and whether 'Edhas' felt more threatened being the only male, as well as the impact on the process of therapy (Goodrich, 1991). When I took the lead, I provoked a conflict in 'Edhas' and adopted a reflexive stance in relation to the power differentials existing within the therapeutic relationship and the family relationships. Circular questioning addressed prejudices, mobilising empathy in the parents towards their daughters' culturally different perspectives on their racial comments about their partners, encouraging them to begin adjusting and accommodating their behaviour accordingly (Laszloffy & Hardy, 2000, p. 37).

I reflected upon gender issues within the context of power and difference and 'Edhas's' extreme vulnerability. I wondered about the relationship between 'Edhas' and 'Aasiya' in terms of the intensity of both having been sexually abused by the same perpetrator. During the middle phase, we discussed distraction techniques to support 'Aasiya's' attempts to regulate her feelings of guilt through obsessional thinking and to soften 'Edhas's' hostile responses to her. By session ten, tension had eased in the family. It transpired that 'Aasiya' reminded 'Edhas' of his abuse, which he wanted to forget, and he wanted for 'Aasiya' to move on. It was considered important to separate their stories, establishing what belongs to whom, alongside that Aasiya was not deliberately being ill.

By session 12, 'Aasiya' requested a session between her and 'Edhas' to address the issue of her lack of protection during childhood. With support from my mentors, I supported 'Aasiya' to utilise the perspective of 'instructive interaction' (Maturana, 1984, p. 246), which 'Edhas' supported, changing the power relations between them. There transpired a sense of co-construction; 'Edhas' listened to 'Aasiya's' narrative, facilitated by previously interviewing 'Edhas's' internal other for increased empathy with 'Aasiya'. I reflected that 'as family therapists, we cannot invent a family' (Cecchin, 1987, p. 3) but, perhaps, facilitate patterns towards new scripts and better stories (Pocock, 1995, pp. 149–173), and I recognised that significant progress had been made by session 16.

It was helpful to bring 'Family A' to a case consultation, where a role-play took place with 'Think Family' in mind, focusing on 'Sanya' and 'Edhas' as older people, and the unresolved issue of care for 'Aasiya', which had become stuck. Following this, 'Sanya' addressed 'Edhas' more directly regarding 'Aasiya's' care.

### Ending and outcomes

This section will illustrate my awareness of how change would be recognised within the therapeutic model(s) being used, including a brief description of the outcome in terms of both individual and family change. An account will also be given of the way issues of ending were addressed in therapy.

The main helpful models of change during this process were associated with the Milan School, mainly following Cecchin's thinking about curiosity, prejudices and tracking beliefs. Significant change occurred through my continued questioning of the beliefs and prejudices of 'Edhas' and 'Sanya', facilitating empathy and supporting 'Aasiya' to have a secure voice in the family. Importantly, I tried to maintain a reflexive stance, considering the relationship between self, other and context, and expanding the frame by examining the underlying assumptions and priorities that shaped interactions. Separating 'Aasiya's' experience of abuse from 'Edhas's' made a significant change to 'Aasiya's' more established place in the family.

I considered that change could take place by accepting 'Family A' as they were, encouraging trust in me and the process and enabling a wider variety of patterns to emerge without *expecting* change. From an aesthetic perspective, this would give different options (Cecchin, 1987, p. 4). Alongside using post-Milan narrative approaches, I also considered the life-cycle model in thinking about transitions. CMM techniques were invaluable for interpreting very difficult interactions.

Following the case consultation, 'Sanya' decided to move to their home out of London by June 2020. 'Sanya' and 'Edhas' decided to obtain psychiatric treatment for 'Aasiya' privately. 'Family A's' request for the family therapy to continue until May 2020 was agreed by the NHS and supported by my mentor as the ending phase to be carefully worked through.

By session 23, 'Aasiya's' difficulties became more of a shared problem, as the parents began to acknowledge these, therefore, taking more responsibility.

A dialogue about abuse was opened up in the family, and 'Sanya', 'Amar', 'Ahmed' and 'Kanesh's' thoughts and feelings were heard, creating a shared sense of grieving. The impact that 'Aasiya' has on 'Edhas' and vice versa was thoroughly explored, with 'Edhas' owning his own history of abuse.

A few months following ending this work, Aasiya contacted me speaking of concerns about family members swapping their identities and being frightened about family not being who they said they were, frightened that they were going to harm her. Aasiya's presentation can be thought about in light of delusional misidentification syndromes, the generic term for the conditions that are characterised by misidentification of close relatives. The individual conditions include Capgras syndrome, Fregoli syndrome, syndromes of intermetamorphosis and subjective doubles and reduplicative paramnesia. Beyond these helpful psychiatric observations, I wondered if Aasiya was inherently and understandably confused through the confusion of family roles becoming sexualised at such a young age and this state of mind being easily triggered in the present in relation to anxieties. In therapy, one is trained not to offer reassurance to clients since reassurance is generally false. However, with the exception of individuals experiencing psychotic-like episodes, such as Aasiya's presentation here, reassurance is exactly what is needed to help contain acute and terrifying states of mind, such as hers.

Aasiya wanted to resume therapy with me, which I offered through individual weekly sessions, supporting her in and out of inpatient hospital wards. Her vulnerability to repeating the sexual abuse of her early life with relative strangers and her seemingly high sexual arousal decreased over time but was a risk. It seemed that her parents had not recognised this as a risk, and her paying people to be friends with her was a further risk in terms of her being financially and emotionally exploited. Trust had been established with Aasiya near the beginning of our professional relationship on the assessment ward, but I further considered this in the context of her propensity to depend on others for her sense of safety and security at a survival level.

Over time, Aasiya started writing about her experiences, at first finding this too exposing, but she then wrote more of her experiences. Aasiya's accounts of her experiences highlight the almost unthinkable suffering reported by individuals with schizophrenia, which is mostly ignored by the majority. Understandably, on the one hand, the experience of paranoia, which takes a person away from reality, can only be one of the most terrifying states of mind to be in, where trust cannot be checked but utter dependence on others is so high a need due to past sexually abusive experiences. The medications offered to individuals such as 'Aasiya' do improve everyday functioning but not enough, perhaps due to a lack of medical understanding of the mind yet. However, being aware of the poor quality of life for individuals such as Aasiya, it is hard to accept that we can surely use our skills, intelligence and knowledge to help improve life for these people, who suffer so exponentially, at no seeming fault of their own.

*Figure 11.1* Big red painting

# Reflections and learning

This section will include my thoughts on what was learnt as a result of this piece of work, considerations of what might have been done differently and aspects that worked well.

The complexity of 'Family A's' difficulties meant that working on my own in their home posed a challenge to remaining in my role due to attempts to absorb me into the family as a friend/carer for 'Aasiya' and as a weapon against the psychiatric system. A main learning point has been the importance of my mentor's support. I learned that it is important not to take full responsibility for the family since 'to take full responsibility for controlling the family problem is to assume that the therapist's job is to instruct', mistakenly assuming a sense of moral superiority, which is limiting and 'masks the ability to be curious about the context' (Cecchin, 1987, p. 4). Maintaining curiosity in myself and the family was difficult but crucial, using the language of relationship by using 'if' and future-oriented questions, which implied patterns not facts (Cecchin, 1987, p. 5).

Remembering my limited power within the family upheld my respect of the system and helped me continue looking for resources within the family. I consider that I have developed as a family therapist in relation to letting go of the need to find a single explanation, helping generating hypotheses (Selvini-Palazzoli et al., 1980, pp. 3–12) and constantly challenging 'family's stories/hypotheses and my stories/hypotheses' (Cecchin, 1987, p. 5), alongside offering constructive feedback and staying with not knowing. Being reflexive has taught me an enormous amount about myself in relation to family therapy through this difficult yet invaluable process.

DOI: 10.4324/9781003509059-13

# Conclusion

My therapeutic work with individuals and families has been an invaluable lifelong source of learning about typical and atypical aspects of the human personality and mind and inevitably about my own sensitivities and strengths. In employing different therapy modalities, I consider that I am communicating that there is enough evidence by now to demonstrate how people with psychosis can be helped in psychotherapy and to encourage many more practitioners to feel equipped to offer spaces in their practices to people with the psychoses and schizophrenias. There appears a lot of fear amongst counsellors and psychotherapists about psychosis. More training clearly needs to be offered about this, and I will, in part, be addressing this need. I must remember that my underpinning philosophy is to give to those who have less than others. People suffering with such changes in reality live in terror of being harmed or harming others and are, in effect, the most vulnerable amongst our communities. They need our help and forbearance since it seems that across all those I have worked with, there is a very vulnerable childhood history, which arrests their development. It also needs to be stated that adopting a pitiful stance towards this population would get us nowhere and having the insight into the methods and mechanisms employed to help such individuals is a necessity. It has been a great pleasure to work with all the individuals that I have met over the last 20 years, working on acute wards and into the community and sometimes back again, navigating the risk. It is difficult to put into words the enormity of what I have and am continuing to learn through the sharings, both individually, in couples and in groups, for which I am immensely grateful. Overall, the Freudian and subsequent Kleinian psychoanalytic thinkers have paved the way for my increased understanding of what may be going on between myself and others in the consulting room, with individuals suffering with the psychoses. However, when individuals are asked if they could live again, whether they would do anything differently, the majority state that they wouldn't want their psychosis changed, due to where it has taken them and what they have learned.

It has also been through close supervision that I have learned to grow and develop in my therapeutic practice with individuals with the psychoses and

DOI: 10.4324/9781003509059-14

intend to continue doing so. My main learning has been that looking beyond and beneath the powerfully obstructive labels of schizophrenia and psychosis, leads to recognising the personality elements that are frequently present amongst this population, namely, paranoid fear, disorganisation, neglect, loss of distinct internal boundaries in relation to the environment and external world, loss of identity, loss of trust in one's perceptions and memory, vulnerability alongside a compulsion to repeat, emotional instability and unexpressed rage and grief. In therapy, each of these elements can be explored with the individual, and a consistent, supportive and reliable routine can be established, from which their lives can start to flourish, as demonstrated in the case studies depicted earlier. Fragile individuals need support to manage the basics in life of: food, water, sleep, communication and exercise, from which over time a more psychodynamic or psychoanalytic approach can gradually be introduced gently and gradually as their ego strength increases. We need to be cautious when individuals start to get better, ensuring they are equally supported through this potentially risky transition in their lives. More people become suicidal in the springtime as the weather gets better and nature starts to flourish. The contrast between the colourful flowers and how some may feel inside themselves can be fatal. The bright flowers, juxtaposed with immense pain and acute grief, can ignite suicidality. Therefore, we need to be very mindful of these more vulnerable people approaching spring and the associated risks, especially those with severe mental health difficulties. I think that the suffering experienced by individuals who are diagnosed with the psychoses and schizophrenias is beyond terrible, and as I have been rightly reminded, 'It's a horrible, horrible, horrible illness – schizophrenia', beyond what I admit I can fully grasp. I further keep in mind the carers of individuals who are suffering, recognising that much more needs to be done to offer support to family members cross-culturally so they feel understood. I am heartened to hear that carer support groups are burgeoning. I aim to keep my consulting room door open to those presenting with psychoses and schizophrenias, their families and carers. More doors need to be opened to welcome and help our fellow humankind, from a place of social justice and peace of mind. The suffering described in the case studies earlier, at such exponential levels, is an ethical issue that needs addressing. All comments, feedback and discussion points, please send to helenholmes009@gmail.com. Thank you for taking the time to read my thoughts.

# References

Adler, R. H. (2009). Engel's biopsychosocial model is still relevant today. *Journal of Psychosomatic Research, 67*(6), 607–611.

Aggett, P., Sainson, M., & Tapsell, D. (2011). 'Seeking permission': An interviewing stance for finding connection with hard to reach families. *Journal of Family Therapy, 37*(2).

Alleyne, A. (2004). The internal oppressor and black identify wounding. *Counselling and Psychotherapy Journal, 15*(10), 48–50.

American Psychiatric Association. (1994). *Diagnostic and statistical manual of mental disorders* (4th ed.). American Psychiatric Association.

American Psychiatric Association. (2013). *Diagnostic and statistical manual of mental disorders* (5th ed.). American Psychiatric Association.

Andersen, T. (1990). *The reflecting team: Dialogue and dialogues about dialogues.* Norton.

Barkham, M., Bewick, B., Mullin, T., Gilbody, S., Connell, J., Cahill, J., & Evans, C. (2013). The CORE-10: A short measure of psychological distress for routine use in the psychological therapies. *Counselling and Psychotherapy Research, 13*(1), 3–13.

Barnes, O. (2024). Schizophrenia: The new drug set to tackle the 'cancer of psychiatry'. *The Financial Times.* https://www.ft.com/content/427d37df-e2e9-4b67-87be-29f2a258de00

Bartholomew, T. F., Pérez-Rojas, A. E., Kang, E., & Joy, E. E. (2020). Refinement and factor structure confirmation of the inventory of therapist work with client assets and strengths (IT-WAS). *Counselling Psychology Quarterly, 33*(4), 448–464.

Bell, D. (2003). *Ideas in psychoanalysis: Paranoia.* Icon Books, Totem Books.

Berg, I. K., & Dolan, Y. (2001). *Tales of solutions: A collection of hope-inspiring stories.* Norton.

Berzlanovich, A. M., Schopfer, J., & Keil, W. (2012). Deaths due to physical restraint. *Deutsches Ärzteblatt International, 109*(3), 27–32.

Bieling, P. J., & Kukyen, W. (2003). Is cognitive case formulation science or science fiction? *Clinical Psychology: Science and Practice, 10*(1), 52–69.

Bion, W. (1955, October 5). *Differentiation of the psychotic from the non-psychotic personalities.* Paper read before the British Psycho-Analytical Society.

Bohart, A. C., & Tallman, K. (1999). The client as a common factor: Clients as self-healers. In M. Hubble, B. L. Duncan, & S. D. Miller (Eds.), *The heart and soul of change: What works in therapy* (pp. 91–131). American Psychological Association.

Bor, R., & Watts, M. (2017). *The trainee handbook: A guide for counselling and psychotherapy trainees* (4th ed.). Sage Publications.

Borras, L., Mohr, S., Brandt, P. Y., Gilliéron, C., Eytan, A., & Huguelet, P. (2007). Religious beliefs in schizophrenia: Their relevance for adherence to treatment. *Schizophrenia Bulletin, 33,* 1238–1246.

Borras, L., Mohr, S., Brandt, P. Y., Gillieron, C., Eytan, A., & Huguelet, P. (2008). Influence of spirituality and religiousness on smoking among patients with schizophrenia or schizo-affective disorder in Switzerland. *International Journal of Social Psychiatry, 54*, 539–549.

Bozarth, J. D. (1998). Person-centered therapy: A revolutionary paradigm. Ross-on-Wye, England: PCCS Books.

Brewerton, T. D. (1994). Hyperreligiosity in psychotic disorders. *Journal of Nervous and Mental Disease, 182*, 302.

British Psychological Society. (2011). *Good practice guidelines on the use of psychological formulation*. British Psychological Society.

British Psychological Society. (2017). *Practice guidelines* (3rd ed.). British Psychological Society.

British Psychological Society. (2020). *Guidance for BPS accredited psychology professional doctorate programmes in relation to the Covid-19 outbreak (2020)*. British Psychological Society. https://www.bps.org.uk/sites/www.bps.org.uk/files/Accreditation/Guidance%20for%20accredited%20psychology%20professional%20doctorate%20programmes.pdf

British Psychological Society. (2021). *Guidance for psychological professionals working in NHS commissioned services in England during the Covid-19 pandemic*. British Psychological Sochttps://www.bps.org.uk/sites/www.bps.org.uk/files/Policy/Policy%20-%20Files/Guidance%20for%20psychological%20professionals%20during%20Covid-19.pdf

Bronfenbrenner, U. (1977). Toward an experimental ecology of human development. *American Psychologist, 32*(7), 513–531.

Buber, M. (1970). *I and thou*. Charles Scribner's Sons.

Byng-Hall, J. (1995). *Rewriting family scripts*. Guilford Press.

Carter, B., & McGoldrick, M. (2004). *The expanded family life-cycle: Individual, family and social perspectives* (3rd ed.). Allyn and Bacon Classics.

Cecchin, G. (1987). Hypothesizing, circularity and neutrality revisited: An invitation to curiosity. *Family Processes, 26*, 405–413.

Challoner, H., & Papayianni, F. (2012). Evaluating the role of formulation in counselling psychology: A systematic literature review. *Journal of Counselling Psychology, 7*(1), 47–68.

Chantler, K. (2005). From disconnection to connection: 'Race', gender and the politics of therapy. *British Journal of Guidance & Counselling, 33*(2), 239–256.

Cohen, C. I., Jimenez, C., & Mittal, S. (2010). The role of religion in the well-being of older adults with schizophrenia. *Psychiatric Services, 61*, 917–922.

Compion, J., & Bhugra, D. (1997). Experiences of religious healing in psychiatric patients in South India. *Social Psychiatry and Psychiatric Epidemiology, 32*, 215–221.

Conrad, R., Schilling, G., Najjar, D., Geiser, F., Sharif, M., & Liedtke, R. (2007). Cross-cultural comparison of explanatory models of illness in schizophrenic patients in Jordan and Germany. *Psycholical Reports, 101*(2), 531–546.

Cook, C. C. H. (2012). Psychiatry in scripture: Sacred texts and psychopathology. *The Psychiatrist, 36*, 225–229.

Cook, J. M., & O'Hara, C. C. (2020). An emerging theory of the persistence of social class microaggressions: An interpretative phenomenological study. *Counselling Psychology Quarterly, 33*(4), 516–540.

Cooper, M. (2000). Person-centred developmental theory: Reflections and revisions. *Person-Centred Practice, 8*(2), 87–94.

Cooper, M. (2009). Welcoming the other: Actualising the humanistic ethic at the core of counselling psychology practice. *Counselling Psychology Review, 24*(3), 119–129.

Cooper, M. (2021). Directionality: Unifying psychological and social understanding of well-being and distress through an existential ontology. *The Journal of Humanistic Counselling, 60*(1), 6–25.

Cooper, M., & Law, D. (2018). *Working with goals in psychotherapy and counselling.* Oxford University Press.

Cooper, M., & Norcross, J. (2021). Working with client preferences. *Therapy Today, 32*(3), 32–35.

Cooper, M., Van Rijn, B., Chryssafidou, E., & Stiles, W. B. (2021). Activity preferences in psychotherapy: What do patients want and how does this relate to outcomes and alliance? *Counselling Psychology Quarterly.* https://doi.org/10.1080/09515070.2021.1877620

Cromby, J., Harper, D., & Reavey, P. (2013). *Psychology, mental health and distress.* Palgrave Macmillan.

Culliford, L. (2002). Spirituality and clinical care. *BMJ, 325*, 1434–1435.

Dazzan, P., Murray, R., & Nettis, M. (2024). Development and initial evaluation of a clinical prediction model for risk of treatment resistance in first-episode psychosis schizophrenia prediction of resistance to treatment. *British Journal of Psychiatry International.*

Dein, S., & Cook, C. C. H. (2015). God put a thought into my mind: The charismatic Christian experience of receiving communications from God. *Mental Health, Religion & Culture*, 1–17.

Dein, S., & Littlewood, R. (2007). The voice of God. *Anthropology & Medicine, 14*, 213–228.

Diamond, M. J. (2020). Return of the repressed: Revisiting dissociation and the psychoanalysis of the traumatized mind. *Journal of the American Psychoanalytic Association, 68*(5), 839–874.

Dudek, A., Krzystanek, M., Krysta, K., & Gorna, A. (2019). Evolution of religious topics in schizophrenia in 80 years period. *Psychiatria Danubina, 31*(3), 524–529. Retrieved April 22, 2024, from https://www.researchgate.net/publication/336776666_Evolution_of_Religious_Topics_in_Schizophrenia_in_80_Years_Period

Eels, T. D. (2007). *Handbook of psychotherapy case formulation.* Guildford Press.

Eels, T. D., & Lombart, K. G. (2003). Case formulation and treatment concepts among novice, experienced, and expert cognitive-behavioural and psychodynamic therapists. *Psychotherapy Research, 13*(2), 187–204.

Elliott, R., & Westwell, G. (2012). *Person-centred & experiential psychotherapy scale-10.* https://moodle.roehampton.ac.uk/pluginfile.php/184990/mod_resource/content/1/PCEPS-10%20v1.2%5Bpdf%5D.pdf

Engel, G. L. (1977). The need for a new medical model: A challenge for biomedicine. *Science, 196*, 129–136.

Field, H., & Waldfogel, S. (1995). Severe ocular self-injury. *General Hospital Psychiatry, 17*, 224–227.

Flics, D. H., & Herron, W. G. (1991). Activity-withdrawal, diagnosis, and demographics as predictors of premorbid adjustment. *Journal of Clinical Psychology, 47*, 189–198.

Flinn, L., Braham, L., & das Nair, R. (2015). How reliable are case formulations? A systematic literature review. *British Journal of Clinical Psychology, 54*, 266–290.

Foucault, M. (1977). *Discipline and punish: The birth of the prison.* Pantheon Books.

Franco, M., Toomey, T., DeBlaere, C., & Rice, K. (2021). Identity incongruent discrimination, racial identity, and mental health for multiracial individuals. *Counselling Psychology Quarterly, 34*(1), 87–108. https://doi.org/10.1080/09515070.2019.1663788

Freeman, T., Cameron, J. L., & McGhie, A. (1958). *Chronic schizophrenia.* Tavistock Publications.

Freire, E. S., Cooper, M., & Elliott, R. (2007). *The Strathclyde inventory: Validation of a person-centred outcome measure.* Paper presented at the 13th Annual BACP Counselling and Psychotherapy Research Conference.

Freud, S. (1896). Further remarks on the neuro-psychoses of defence. In *The standard edition III, the complete psychological works of Sigmund Freud*. Hogarth Press.

Freud, S. (1901). The psychopathology of everyday life. In *The complete psychological works of Sigmund Freud*. Hogarth Press.

Freud, S. (1914). Remembering, repeating and working-through (further recommendations on the technique of psycho-analysis II). In *The standard edition of the complete psychological works of Sigmund Freud* (Vol. 12, pp. 145–156). Hogarth Press.

Freud, S. (1917). Mourning and melancholia. In J. Strachey (Ed.), *The standard edition of the complete psychological works of Sigmund Freud, Vol. XIV, 1914–1916, 1953*. Hogarth Press.

Gaite, L., Vázquez-Barquero, J. L., Borra, C., Ballesteros, J., Schene, A., Welcher, B., Thornicroft, G., Becker, T., Ruggeri, M., Herran, A., & EPSILON Study Group. (2002). Quality of life in patients with schizophrenia in five European countries: The EPSILON study. *Acta Psychiatrica Scandinavica, 105*, 283–292.

Gearing, R. E., Alonzo, D., Smolak, A., McHugh, K., Harmon, S., & Baldwin, S. (2011). Association of religion with delusions and hallucinations in the context of schizophrenia: Implications for engagement and adherence. *Schizophrenia Research, 126*, 150–163.

Geller, S. M. (2013). Therapeutic presence: An essential way of being. In M. Cooper, P. F. Schmid, M. O' Hara, & A. C. Bohart (Eds.), *The handbook of person-centred psychotherapy and counselling* (2nd ed., pp. 209–222). Palgrave Macmillan.

Geller, S. M., Greenberg, L. S., & Watson, J. C. (2010). Therapist and client perceptions of therapeutic presence: The development of a measure, *Psychotherapy Research, 20*(5), 599–610.

Gendlin, E. T. (1964). A theory of personality change. In P. Worchel & D. Byrne (Eds.), *Personality change* (pp. 100–148). John Wiley & Sons.

Gendlin, E. T. (1981). *Focusing* (2nd ed.). Bantam Books.

Gendlin, E. T., & Zimring, F. (1955). *The qualities or dimensions of experiencing and their change* (Counseling Center Discussion Papers, 1, 3). University of Chicago Library.

General Data Protection Regulation. (2020). *European parliament and council of the European Union*. https://gdpr-info.eu/

Gergen, K. J., Hoffman, L., & Anderson, H. (1996). Is diagnosis a disaster? A constructionist trialogue. In F. Kaslow (Ed.), *Relational diagnosis*. Wiley & Sons.

Gersch, E., Leimaa, M., Hulbert, C., McCutcheon, L., Burke, E., Valkonen, H., Tikkanen, S., & Chanen, A. M. (2018). Alliance rupture and repair processes in borderline personality disorder; a case study using dialogical sequence analysis. *Counselling Psychology Quarterly, 31*(4), 477–496.

Gilligan, C. (1982). *In a different voice: Psychological theory and women's development*. Harvard University Press.

Gillon, E. (2012). A response to Simms (2011): Case formulation within a person-centred framework: An uncomfortable fit? *Counselling Psychology Review, 27*(1), 73–76.

Goodman, L. A., Liang, B., Helms, J. E., Latta, R. E., Sparks, E., & Weintraub, S. R. (2004). Training counselling psychologists as social justice agents: Feminist and multicultural principles in action. *The Counseling Psychologist, 32*(6), 793–837.

Goodrich, T. J. (1991). *Women and power: Perspectives for family therapy*. W. W. Norton.

Goss, D. (2016). Integrating neuroscience into counselling psychology: A systematic review of current literature. *The Counselling Psychologist, 44*(6), 895–920.

Greenberg, D., & Brom, D. (2001). Nocturnal hallucinations in ultra-orthodox Jewish Israeli men. *Psychiatry, 64*, 81–89.

Groth-Marnat, G. (2003). *Handbook of psychological assessment* (4th ed.). John Wiley & Sons.

Health and Care Professions Council. (2015). *Standards of proficiency: Practitioner psychologists.* Health and Care Professions Council. https://www.hcpc-uk.org/standards/standards-of-proficiency/practitioner-psychologists/

Herman, J. (2015). *Trauma and recovery: From domestic abuse to political terror.* Pandora.

Holmes, H. (2020). *Seeing God in our birth experiences: A psychoanalytic inquiry into pre and perinatal religious development.* Routledge Books.

Horvath, A. O., & Greenberg, L. S. (Eds.). (1994). *Wiley series on personality processes. The working alliance: Theory, research, and practice.* John Wiley & Sons.

Huang, C. L., Shang, C. Y., Shieh, M. S., Lin, H. N., & Su, J. C. (2011). The interactions between religion, religiosity, religious delusion/hallucination, and treatment-seeking behavior among schizophrenic patients in Taiwan. *Psychiatry Research, 187,* 347–353.

Huguelet, P., Binyet-Vogel, S., Gonzalez, C., Favre, S., & McQuillan, A. (1997). Follow-up study of 67 first episode schizophrenic patients and their involvement in religious activities. *European Psychiatry, 12,* 279–283.

Huguelet, P., Borras, L., Gillieron, C., Brandt, P. Y., & Mohr, S. (2009). Influence of spirituality and religiousness on substance misuse in patients with schizophrenia or schizo-affective disorder. *Substance Use & Misuse, 44,* 502–513.

Huguelet, P., Mohr, S., Borras, L., Gillieron, C., & Brandt, P. Y. (2006). Spirituality and religious practices among outpatients with schizophrenia and their clinicians. *Psychiatric Services, 57,* 366–372.

Huguelet, P., Mohr, S., Jung, V., Gillieron, C., Brandt, P. Y., & Borras, L. (2007). Effect of religion on suicide attempts in outpatients with schizophrenia or schizo-affective disorders compared with inpatients with non-psychotic disorders. *European Psychiatry, 22,* 188–194.

Husserl, E. (1969). *Ideas: General introduction to pure phenomenology.* George Allen & Unwin.

Johnson, S., Sathyaseelan, M., Charles, H., Jeyaseelan, V., & Jacob, K. S. (2012). Insight, psychopathology, explanatory models and outcome of schizophrenia in India: A prospective 5-year cohort study. *BMC Psychiatry, 12,* 159.

Johnstone, L., & Boyle, M. (2018). The power-threat meaning framework: An alternative nondiagnostic conceptual system. *Journal of Humanistic Counseling,* 1–18.

Johnstone, L., Boyle, M., Cromby, J., Dillon, J., Harper, D., Kinderman, P., Longden, E., Pilgrim, D., & Read, J. (2018). *The power threat meaning framework: Towards the identification of patterns in emotional distress, unusual experiences and troubled or troubling behaviour, as an alternative to functional psychiatric diagnosis.* British Psychological Society.

Johnstone, L., Boyle, M., Cromby, J., Dillon, J., Harper, D., Kinderman, P., Longden, E., Pilgrim, D., & Read, J. (2019). Reflections on responses to the power threat meaning framework one year on. *Clinical Psychology Forum, 313.*

Johnstone, L., & Dallos, R. (2014). *Formulation in psychology and psychotherapy: Making sense of people's problems.* Routledge.

Joseph, S., & Worsley, R. (2005). *Person-centred psychopathology: A positive psychology of mental health* (pp. 348–357). PCCS Books.

Kagan, C., Burron, M., Duckett, P., Lawthom, R., & Sidiquee, A. (2011). *Critical community psychology: Critical action and social change.* BPS Blackwell for Wiley & Sons.

Kate, N., Grover, S., Kulhara, P., & Nehra, R. (2012). Supernatural beliefs, aetiological models and help seeking behaviour in patients with schizophrenia. *Industrial Psychiatry Journal, 21,* 49–54.

Kelly, G., Maimon, J., & Scott, J. (1987). Utility of the health belief model in examining medication compliance among psychiatric outpatients. *Social Science & Medicine, 25,* 1205–1211.

Kent, G., & Wahass, S. (1996). The content and characteristics of auditory hallucinations in Saudi Arabia and the UK: A cross-cultural comparison. *Acta Psychiatrica Scandinavica, 94,* 433–437.

Kirov, G., Kemp, R., Kirov, K., & David, A. S. (1998). Religious faith after psychotic illness. *Psychopathology, 31,* 234–245.

Klein, M. H., Mathieu, P. L., Gendlin, E. T., & Kiesler, D. J. (1969). *The experiencing scale: A research and training manual* (Vol. 1). University of Wisconsin Extension Bureau of Audio-Visual Instruction.

Koenig, H. (1990). *Handbook of religion and mental health.* Academic Press.

Kraya, N. A., & Patrick, C. (1997). Folie à deux in forensic setting. *Australian and New Zealand Journal of Psychiatry, 31,* 883–888.

Kroenke, K., Spitzer, R. L., & Williams, J. B. (2001). The PHQ-9: Validity of a brief depression severity measure. *Journal of General Internal Medicine, 16*(9), 606–613.

Kroll, J., & Sheehan, W. (1989). Religious beliefs and practices among 52 psychiatric inpatients in Minnesota. *The American Journal of Psychiatry, 146,* 67–72.

Krzystanek, M., Krysta, K., Klasik, A., & Krupka-Matuszczyk, I. (2012). Religious content of hallucinations in paranoid schizophrenia. *Psychiatria Danubina, 24*(Suppl 1), S65–S69.

Kuipers, E. (2006). Family interventions in schizophrenia: Evidence for efficacy and proposed mechanisms of change. Journal of Family Therapy, *28*(1), 73–80.

Kulhara, P., Avasthi, A., & Sharma, A. (2000). Magico-religious beliefs in schizophrenia: A study from North India. *Psychopathology, 33,* 62–68.

Lang, W. P., Little, M., & Cronen, V. (1990). The systemic professional: Domains of action and the question of neutrality. *Human Systems, 1,* 32–47.

Laslo-Roth, R., George-Levi, S., & Margalit, M. (2021). Hope during the COVID-19 outbreak: Coping with the psychological impact of quarantine, *Counselling Psychology Quarterly.* https://doi.org/10.1080/09515070.2021.1881762

Laszloffy, T. A., & Hardy, K. V. (2000). Uncommon strategies for a common problem: Addressing racism in family therapy. *Family Process, 39*(1), 35–50.

Lipowski, Z. J. (1989). Psychiatry: Mindless or brainless, both or neither? *The Canadian Journal of Psychiatry, 34,* 249–254.

Littlewood, R., & Lipsedge, M. (1981). Acute psychotic reactions in Caribbean-born patients. *Psychological Medicine, 11,* 303–318.

Lucas, R. (2009). *The psychotic wavelength: A psychoanalytic perspective for psychiatry.* Routledge, Taylor & Francis Group.

Luhrmann, T. M. (2012). *When God talks back.* Knopf.

Macneil, C. A., Hasty, M. K., Conus, P., & Berk, M. (2012). Is diagnosis enough to guide interventions in mental health? Using case formulation in clinical practice. *British Medical Council Medicine, 10*(111), 1–3.

Marley, B., & The Wailers. (1977). *One love, people get ready.* Exodus, Island Records.

Maturana, H. (1984). *Bringing forth of reality.* Presentation at the Family Therapy Program, University of Calgary Medical School.

McClelland, L. (2014). Reformulating the impact of social inequalities. In L. Johnstone & R. Dallos (Eds.), *Formulation in psychology and psychotherapy: Making sense of people's problems* (2nd ed., pp. 121–144). Routledge.

McGoldrick, M., Gerson, R., & Petry, S. (2008). *Genogram: Assessment and intervention.* W.W. Norton.

Mearns, D., & Cooper, M. (2005). *Working at relational depth in counselling and psychotherapy.* Sage.

Mearns, D., & Cooper, M. (2018). *Working at relational depth in counselling and Psychotherapy* (2nd ed.). Sage Publications.

Mearns, D., & Thorne, B. (2000). *Person-centred therapy today: New frontiers in theory and practice.* Sage.

The Mental Capacity Act. (2005). *Legislation.gov.uk*. https://www.legislation.gov.uk/ukpga/2005/9/contents

Mental Health Act. (1983). *legislation.gov.uk*. https://www.legislation.gov.uk/ukpga/1983/20/contents

Mental Health Units (Use of Force) Act. (2018). *Statutory guidance for NHS organisations in England and police forces in England and Wales*. https://www.gov.uk/government/publications/mental-health-units-use-of-force-act-2018

Menzies-Lyth, I. (1988). *Containing anxiety in institutions: Selected essays*. Free Association Books.

Minuchin, S., Rosman, B. L., & Baker, L. (1978). *Psychosomatic families: Anorexia nervosa in context*. Harvard University Press.

Mohr, S., Borras, L., Betrisey, C., Pierre-Yves, B., Gilliéron, C., & Huguelet, P. (2010). Delusions with religious content in patients with psychosis: How they interact with spiritual coping. *Psychiatry, 73*, 158–172.

Mohr, S., Borras, L., Nolan, J., Gillieron, C., Brandt, P. Y., Eytan, A., Leclerc, C., Perroud, N., Whetten, K., Pieper, C., & Koenig, H. G. (2012). Spirituality and religion in outpatients with schizophrenia: A multi-site comparative study of Switzerland, Canada, and the United States. *International Journal of Psychiatry in Medicine, 44*, 29–52.

Mohr, S., Brandt, P. Y., Borras, L., Gilliéron, C., & Huguelet, P. (2006). Toward an integration of spirituality and religiousness into the psychosocial dimension of schizophrenia. *American Journal of Psychiatry, 163*, 1952–1959.

Mohr, S., Ho, J., Duffecy, J., Baron, K. G., Lehmann, K. A., Jin, L., & Reifler, D. (2007). *Journal of Clinical Psychology, 66*(4), 394–409.

Mohr, S., & Huguelet, P. (2004). The relationship between schizophrenia and religion and its implications for care. *Swiss Medical Weekly, 134*, 369–376.

Mohr, S., Perroud, N., Gillieron, C., Brandt, P. Y., Rieben, I., Borras, L., & Huguelet, P. (2011). Spirituality and religiousness as predictive factors of outcome in schizophrenia and schizo-affective disorders. *Psychiatry Research, 186*, 177–182.

Mumma, G. (2011). Validity issues in cognitive-behavioural case formulation. *European Journal of Psychological Assessment, 27*(1), 29–49.

Mundt, J. C., Marks, I. M., Shear, M. K., & Griest, J. H. (2002). The work and social adjustment scale: A simple measure of impairment in functioning. *British Journal of Psychiatry, 180*, 461–464.

Murray-Swank, A., Goldberg, R., Dickerson, F., Medoff, D., Wohlheiter, K., & Dixon, L. (2007). Correlates of religious service attendance and contact with religious leaders among persons with co-occurring serious mental illness and type 2 diabetes. *The Journal of Nervous and Mental Disease, 195*, 382–388.

Napo, F., Heinz, A., & Auckenthaler, A. (2012). Explanatory models and concepts of West African Malian patients with psychotic symptoms. *European Psychiatry, 27*(Suppl 2), S44–S49.

National Institute of Clinical Excellence (NICE). (2007). *Depression (amended): Management of depression in primary and secondary care*. National Institute for Clinical Excellence.

Neeleman, J., & Lewis, G. (1994). Religious identity and comfort beliefs in three groups of psychiatric patients and a group of medical controls. *International Journal of Social Psychiatry, 40*, 124.

Neimeyer, R. A., Klass, D., & Dennis, M. R. (2014). A social constructionist account of grief: Loss and the narration of meaning. *Death Studies, 38*, 485–498.

Nolan, J. A., McEvoy, J. P., Koenig, H. G., Hooten, E. G., Whetten, K., & Pieper, C. F. (2012). Religious coping and quality of life among individuals living with schizophrenia. *Psychiatric Services, 63*, 1051–1054.

Nurasikin, M. S., Khatijah, L. A., Aini, A., Ramli, M., Aida, S. A., Zainal, N. Z., & Ng, C. G. (2013). Religiousness, religious coping methods and distress level among psychiatric patients in Malaysia. *International Journal of Social Psychiatry*, *59*, 332–338.

Orlans, V., & Van Scoyoc, S. (2008). *A short introduction to counselling psychology*. Google Books. https://books.google.co.uk/books?id=jqP5HGzw8MC&printsec=frontcover &dq=counselling+psychology&hl=en&sa=X&ved=0ahUKEwja49_e0dPSAhUEI8A KHasfDeEQ6AEIJDAC#v=onepage&q=counselling%20psychology&f=false>

Padmavati, R., Thara, R., & Corin, E. (2005). A qualitative study of religious practices by chronic mentally ill and their caregivers in South India. *International Journal of Social Psychiatry*, *51*, 139–149.

Palazolli, M. S., Boscolo, L., Cecchin, G., & Prata, G. (1980). The problem of the referring person. *Journal of Marital and Family Therapy*, *6*(1), 3–9.

Palazzoli S, M., Boscolo, L., Cecchin, G., & Prata, G. (1980). Hypothesizing — Circularity — Neutrality: Three Guidelines for the Conductor of the Session. *Journal of Family Process*, *19*(1), 3–12.

Pargament, K. I., Koenig, H. G., & Perez, L. M. (2000). The many methods of religious coping: Development and initial validation of the RCOPE. *Journal of Clinical Psychology*, *56*, 519–543.

Pearce, W. B. (2005). The co-ordinated management of meaning. In W. B. Gudykunst (Ed.), *Theorizing about intercultural communication*. Sage Publications.

Peters, E., Day, S., McKenna, J., & Orbach, G. (1999). Delusional ideation in religious and psychotic populations. *British Journal of Clinical Psychology*, *38*, 83–96.

Phillips, R., & Stein, C. (2007). God's will, God's punishment, or God's limitations? Religious coping strategies reported by young adults living with serious mental illness. *Journal of Clinical Psychology*, *63*, 529–540.

Pieper, J. Z. (2004). Religious coping in highly religious psychiatric inpatients. *Mental Health, Religion & Culture*, *7*, 349–363.

Pocock, D. (1995). Searching for a better story: Harnessing modern and postmodern positions in family therapy. *Journal of Family Therapy*, *17*, 149–173.

Reddy, W. M. (2020). The unavoidable intentionality of affect: The history of emotions and the neurosciences of the present day. *Emotion Review*, *12*(3), 168–178.

Reger, G. M., & Rogers, S. A. (2002). Diagnostic differences in religious coping among individuals with persistent mental illness. *Journal of Psychology and Christianity*, *21*(3), 41–48.

Revheim, N., Greenberg, W. M., & Citrome, L. (2010). Spirituality, schizophrenia, and state hospitals: Program description and characteristics of self-selected attendees of a spirituality therapeutic group. *Psychiatric Quarterly*, *81*, 285–292.

Rey, H. (1994). *Universals of psychoanalysis in the treatment of psychotic and borderline states: Factors of space-time and language* (J. Magagna, Ed.). Free Association Books.

Rogers, C. R. (1942). *Counseling and psychotherapy: Newer concepts in practice*. Houghton Mifflin.

Rogers, C. R. (1951). *Client-centred therapy*. Constable and Robinson Ltd.

Rogers, C. R. (1956). Client-centred theory. *Journal of Counseling Psychology*, *3*(2), 115–120.

Rogers, C. R. (1957). The necessary ad sufficient conditions of therapeutic personality change. *Journal of Consulting Psychology*, *21*(2), 95–103.

Rogers, C. R. (1958). A process conception of psychotherapy. *American Psychologist*, *13*, 142–149.

Rogers, C. R. (1959). Theory of therapy, personality and interpersonal relationships as developed in the client-centered framework. In S. Koch (Ed.), *Psychology: A study of a science, formulations of the person and the social context* (Vol. 3, pp. 184–256). McGraw Hill.

Rogers, C. R. (1960). Significant trends in the client-centred orientation. In D. Brower & L. E. Abt (Eds.), *Progress in clinical psychology* (Vol. IV). Grune & Stratton.

Rogers, C. R. (1961a). *On becoming a person: A therapist's view of psychotherapy*. Constable.

Rogers, C. R. (1961b). The process equation of psychotherapy. *American Journal of Psychotherapy, 15,* 27–45.

Rogers, C. R. (1973). The interpersonal relationship; the core of guidance. In C. R. Rogers & B. Stevens (Eds.), *Person to person: The problem of being human* (pp. 89–103). Souvenir Press.

Rogers, C. R. (1979). The foundations of the person-centred approach. *Education, 100*(2), 98–107.

Rogers, C. R. (1980a). *A way of being.* Houghton Mifflin.

Rogers, C. R. (1980b). *Client-centred psychotherapy* (H. I. Kaplan, A. M. Freedman, & B. J. Sadock, Eds., Vol. II, 3rd ed., pp. 2153–2168). Williams and Wilkins.

Rogers, C. R. (1992). The necessary and sufficient conditions of therapeutic personality change. *Journal of Consulting and Clinical Psychology, 60*(6), 827–832.

Rogers, C. R. (2002). Reflection of feelings. In D. J. Cain (Ed.), *Classics in the person-centred approach* (pp. 13–14). PCCS Books.

Rogers, C. R., Gendlin, E. T., Kiesler, D. J., & Truax, C. B. (1967). *The therapeutic relationship and its impact: A study of psychotherapy with schizophrenics.* Greenwood Press.

Rogers, C. R., & Rablen, R. A. (1958). *A scale of process in psychotherapy.* University of Wisconsin.

Rosenfeld, H. (1971). A clinical approach to the psychoanalytical theory of the life and death instincts: An investigation into the aggressive aspects of narcissism. *International Journal of Psychoanalysis, 52,* 169–178.

Rosenfeld, H. (1988). *Impasse and interpretation: Therapeutic and anti-therapeutic factors in the psychoanalytic treatment of psychotic, borderline and neurotic patients. The new library of psychoanalysis.* Routledge.

Rudaleviciene, P., Stompe, T., Narbekovas, A., Raskauskiene, N., & Bunevicius, R. (2008). Are religious delusions related to religiosity in schizophrenia? *Medicina (Kaunas), 44,* 529–535.

Rund, B. R. (1990). Fully recovered schizophrenics: A retrospective study of some premorbid and treatment factors. *Psychiatry, 53,* 127–139.

Safran, J. D., Muran, J. C., & Eubanks-Carter, C. (2011). Repairing alliance ruptures. In J. C. Norcross (Ed.), *Psychotherapy relationships that work: Evidence-based responsiveness* (2nd ed., pp. 224–238). Oxford University Press.

Sanders, P. (2005). Principled and strategic opposition to the medicalisation of distress and all of its apparatus. In S. Joseph & R. Worsley (Eds.), *Person-centred psychopathology: A positive psychology of mental health* (pp. 21–42). PCCS Books.

Saravanan, B., Jacob, K. S., Deepak, M. G., Prince, M., David, A. S., & Bhugra, D. (2008). Perceptions about psychosis and psychiatric services: A qualitative study from Vellore, India. *Social Psychiatry and Psychiatric Epidemiology, 43,* 231–238.

Saravanan, B., Jacob, K. S., Johnson, S., Prince, M., Bhugra, D., & David, A. S. (2007). Belief models in first episode schizophrenia in South India. *Social Psychiatry and Psychiatric Epidemiology, 42,* 446–451.

Schmid, P. F. (2006). The challenge of the other: Towards dialogical person-centred psychotherapy and counselling. *Person-Centred & Experiential Psychotherapies, 5*(4), 240–254.

Schmidt, S. (2009). Shall we really do it again? The powerful concept of replication is neglected in the social sciences. *Review of General Psychology, 13*(2), 90–100.

Shah, R., Kulhara, P., Grover, S., Kumar, S., Malhotra, R., & Tyagi, S. (2011a). Relationship between spirituality/religiousness and coping in patients with residual schizophrenia. *Quality of Life Research, 20,* 1053–1060.

Shah, R., Kulhara, P., Grover, S., Kumar, S., Malhotra, R., & Tyagi, S. (2011b). Contribution of spirituality to quality of life in patients with residual schizophrenia. *Psychiatry Research, 190,* 200–205.

Siddle, R., Haddock, G., Tarrier, N., & Faragher, E. B. (2002). Religious delusions in patients admitted to hospital with schizophrenia. *Social Psychiatry and Psychiatric Epidemiology, 37*, 130–138.

Simms, J. (2011). Case formulation within a person-centred framework; An uncomfortable fit? *Counselling Psychology Review, 26*, 24–36.

Smith, S., & Suto, M. J. (2012). Religious and/or spiritual practices: Extending spiritual freedom to people with schizophrenia. *Canadian Journal of Occupational Therapy, 79*, 77–85.

Spinelli, E. (2005). *The interpreted world: An introduction to phenomenological psychology.* Sage.

Spinelli, E. (2014). An existential challenge to some dominant perspectives in the practice of contemporary counselling psychology. Counselling Psychology Review, *29*(2), 7–14.

Spitzer, R. L., Kroenke, K., Williams, J. B. W., & Bernd Lowe, D. S. W. (2006, May 22). A brief measure for assessing generalized anxiety disorder: The GAD-7. *Archives of International Medicine, 166*(10), 1092–1097.

Steiner, J. (2012). *Henri Rey, Melanie Klein trust.* https://melanie-klein-trust.org.uk/writers/henri-rey/

Stier, M., Muders, S., Rüther, M., & Schöne-Seifert, B. (2013). Biologismus-Kontroversen – Ethische Implikationen fur die Psychiatrie. *Der Nervenarzt, 10*, 1165–1174.

Stier, M., Schoene-Seifert, B., Ruther, M., & Muders, S. (2014). The philosophy of psychiatry and biologism. *Frontiers in Psychology, 5*, 1–3.

Temaner, B. S. (1977). *The empathic understanding response process.* Chicago Counseling and Psychotherapy Center.

Tepper, L., Rogers, S. A., Coleman, E. M., & Malony, H. N. (2001). The prevalence of religious coping among persons with persistent mental illness. *Psychiatric Services, 52*, 660–665.

Tronick, E. Z., & Weinberg, M. K. (1997). Depressed mothers and infants: Failure to form dyadic states of consciousness. In L. Murray & P. J. Cooper (Eds.), *Postpartum depression and child development* (pp. 54–81). Guilford Press.

Tufekcioglu, S., & Muran, C. (2015). Case formulation and the therapeutic relationship: The role of therapist self-reflection and self-revelation. *Journal of Clinical Psychology: In Session, 71*(5), 469–477.

UK General Data Protection Regulation (UK GDPR, 2025) Available at: https://www.legislation.gov.uk/eur/2016/679/contents

Unal, S., Kaya, B., & Yalvaç, H. D. (2007, Spring). Patients' explanation models for their illness and help-seeking behavior. *Türk Psikiyatri Dergisi, 18*, 38–47.

Van Werde, D., & Prouty, G. (2007). Pre-therapy. In M. Cooper, M. O'Hara, P. F. Schmid, & G. Wyatt (Eds.), *The Handbook of person-centred psychotherapy and counselling* (pp. 237–50). Palgrave Macmillan.

Warner, M. S. (2013). Difficult client process. In M. Cooper, M. O'Hara, P. F. Schmid, & A. C. Bohart (Eds.), *The handbook of person-centred psychotherapy and counselling* (2nd ed., pp. 343–349). Palgrave Macmillan.

Webb, M., Charbonneau, A. M., McCann, R. A., & Gayle, K. R. (2011). Struggling and enduring with God, religious support, and recovery from severe mental illness. *Journal of Clinical Psychology, 67*, 1161–1176.

Wechsler, D. (1997). *Wechsler memory scale-third edition: Administration and scoring manual.* Psychological Corporation, Harcourt Brace & Company.

Weerasekera, P. (1996). *Multiperspective case-formulation: A step towards treatment integration.* Krieger.

White, M., & Epston, D. (1990). *Narrative means to therapeutic ends.* Norton.

Wiggins, S., Elliott, R., & Cooper, M. (2012). The prevalence and characteristics of relational depth events in psychotherapy. *Psychotherapy Research, 22*(2), 139–158.

Wilkins, P., & Gill, M. (2003). Assessment in person-centered therapy. *Person-Centered & Experiential Psychotherapies, 2*(3), 172–187.

Woolfe, R. (1996). The nature of counselling psychology. In R. Woolfe & W. Dryden (Eds.), *Handbook of counselling psychology* (pp. 3–20). Sage.

World Health Organization. (1977). *Manual of the international statistical classification of diseases, injuries, and causes of death (ICD-10)*. Geneva, World Health Organization.

World Health Organization (WHO). (1993). *The ICD-10 classification of mental and behavioural disorders*. World Health Organization.

World Health Organisation. (2019). *International classification of diseases, Eleventh revision (ICD-11)*. World Health Organization (WHO).

Yang, C. T., Narayanasamy, A., & Chang, S. L. (2012). Transcultural spirituality: The spiritual journey of hospitalized patients with schizophrenia in Taiwan. *Journal of Advanced Nursing, 68*, 358–367.

Zahavi, D. (2018). *The Oxford handbook of the history of phenomenology*. Oxford University Press.

Zimmerman, T. S. (2001). *Integrating gender and culture family therapy training*. Haworth Press.

# Index

# Index